I Will Get By

Fred Cadden

Copyright © 2024

All rights reserved.

All rights reserved by Mocha Mint Publishing and Mahogany Ann. No part of this publication may be reproduced, distributed, or transmitted in any form or by any means, including photocopying, recording, or other electronic or mechanical methods, without the author's prior written permission, except in the case of brief quotations embodied in critical reviews and certain other non-commercial uses permitted by copyright law.

Contents

Dedication i
Acknowledgments ii
About the Author iii
Chapter I 1
Chapter II Cam Ranh Bay, Republic of Vietnam 1971 – 1972 17
Chapter III England: 10th Tactical Reconnaissance Wing RAF Alconbury 1972-1975 35
Chapter IV Peaceholme 39
Chapter V Houston, Texas – The Early Years 47
Chapter VI Devastation and Heartbreak 55
Chapter VII Retail Credit at Joske's of Houston 63
Chapter VIII (Oil and Gas Credit) 70
Chapter IX Damson Oil Corporation (1982-1985) 82
Chapter X My Blended Family 89
Chapter XI Apache Corporation (1997 -2019) 99
Chapter XII Enron 101
Chapter XIII Hurricane Katrina (2005) 109
Chapter XIV Reflections 117
Chapter XV Retirement 123
Chapter XVI 129

Dedication

I want to dedicate this book to my children and grandchildren

And to the Memory of my Friend Bennie Sanders

Acknowledgments

My Father, Jack Cadden

My Mother Ida Mae De Lor Cadden

All Close Relatives contributed to my life

Brother Jack

Brother Mike

About the Author

Fred Cadden grew up in the Town of Poughkeepsie, NY, bordering on the Town of Hyde Park, NY, home of FDR. Fred attended Franklin Delano Roosevelt High School, graduating in 1969. He attended Dutchess Community College.

Fred joined the Air Force in 1971. Served in Vietnam 1971-1972. Served in England 1972-1975. Trained as a Medic and Medical Administration.

After the Air Force, Fred moved to Houston, TX, where a summer job was waiting for him. Fred attended the University of Houston from 1975-1977.

Fred worked at Joske's of Houston (now Dillards). Starting out in the Credit Department and working his way up to Assistant Collection Manager.

From there, Fred worked at several Independent Oil and Gas Exploration Companies, where he established the Credit function for the collection of Joint Interest Billings. Fred graduated from The University of Houston Downtown in 1996 With a BBA concentration in Accounting.

Fred is now retired and living in Florida.

Chapter I

I was born in Rhinebeck, NY, to my father, Jack Cadden and my mother, Ida Mae De Lor March 9th, 1951.

I was a premature baby and was kept in an incubator for three months. In 1951, you can imagine how primitive incubators were, and I was called little Freddie under glass by my family. My parents brought me home to our house In Poughkeepsie, New York. This was a house that my great-grandfather had built when he came from Sicily in the late 1800s. It was a three-story house for three families. Each of the children that married would live on each level according to their priority in marriage. Growing up in that house was a loving and nurturing atmosphere and one that I will never forget and always cherish.

Christmas and birthdays are always special occasions that fill my heart with joy and happiness. One could not ask for a better environment, even though my father was a strict disciplinarian. He was firm and always got his point across whenever you screwed up. My mother was the sweetest woman you could ever imagine. She was very religious, and I was raised in the Catholic religion. Everyone who knew my mother respected her and could instantly see her love and caring disposition. She was just a perfect mother to us kids.

Christmas was always a very special time of year. My Grandmother would have all different assortments of candies, cookies, cakes, and pies. I especially enjoyed ribbon candy and the ones with raspberry filling. I remember looking out the frosted windows at the candle decorations, just waiting for Santa to appear that evening. I always loved watching Scrooge, A Christmas Carol by Charles Dickens starring Alistair Simms every night before Christmas on The Million Dollar Movie that ran all week long.

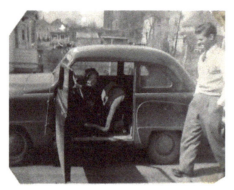

Me and Dad, 1953

I guess I was the favorite of my grandmother until she passed away in 1962. Nanny, as I called her, would spoil me. With my

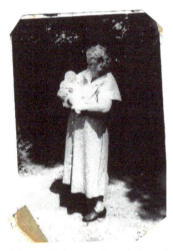

parents living on the second floor, many times I would stay with her overnight on the first floor. Our Family, in the Old-World tradition, was inseparable. I miss her, and I can feel her presence still to this day. I know she's here and pops in and out, and she lets me know she's watching over me. I hope that when I finally move on to the next life, she is waiting for me to guide me into that wonderful realm of heaven.

Me and Nanny, Creek Road

School years are basically uneventful; however, I do remember my first day in First Grade riding the bus to school. I was having such a good time riding on the bus I never got off at my stop, and the bus went back to the school, where they called my parents to come pick me up.

My high school years were challenging, to say the least. I was always a shy guy around girls, so I didn't have many girlfriends. My childhood playmate was my cousin Nancy. We grew up together basically like brother and sister although we were cousins. Our mothers were sisters, and they were very close. My mother and aunt Shirley would get together often during the week and on the weekends, which gave me the joy of being with my cousin who was 2 years older and I looked up to. We would either go adventuring or, in the wintertime, go to her basement and play board games.

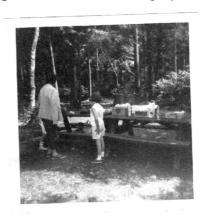

Aunt Shirley Buttonball

I remember going to Nancy's house every other Sunday, and we would watch Dobie Gillis and, later that night, Uncle George's favorite Bonanza. They always had snacks, potato chips, dips or pizza, and Uncle George's Garden always provided fresh tomatoes and vegetables, which were unbelievably delicious. Nanny's favorite show was Gunsmoke, so to this day, I play it in her honor even though I've seen episodes many times. I hope she's watching.

Ever since I can remember, we would go to Buttonball Rest (as Aunt Shirley dubbed it). Initially, it was just a few acres on Wappingers' Creek in Pleasant Valley, NY. We would go on weekends, and in summer, my mother would take us there during the week for a cool, refreshing dip in the 50-degree creek water. I would fish for trout at the rapids that formed from Uncle Georges' makeshift dam and swim down at the deep hole. I loved it there. It was a great getaway and where I learned much about the outdoors. Uncle George purchased the property in the 1950s for $500, and he partnered with his neighbor and friend in Hyde Park. It was only a couple of acres at first, but they expanded it to several acres. Being in the woods and fishing was a great reprise from school and an awesome learning experience that would help me in my scouting endeavors. I miss all that has passed before me. God has blessed me with a good family.

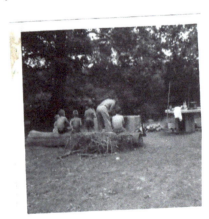

Buttonball

Growing up in my grandparents' house until I was about 10 years old was exceptional. My uncle lived on the first floor with nanny and grandpa, and he had a Television and Radio repair shop on the third floor. We always had a TV for as long as I can remember. When Uncle Bus came home from World War II, he enrolled in the TV in radio repair business school and opened his own shop upon completion. I recall one day, I was probably about 8 years old, and Uncle Bus called me out to the back porch where he had a shortwave radio, and as we looked up into a beautiful starlit sky, we could see Sputnik going across the heavens. Listening to the radio, you could hear the continuous beep, beep, beep from Sputnik. That was the coolest thing I had ever experienced, and it spiked my interest in electronics. I always had either radios or record players and, up until recently, built my own computers. I got in on the ground floor of computers, firstly with the TI4 and then a Commodore 64, then the Apple II, and I just graduated on and on from there.

I remember watching The Beatles on the Ed Sullivan Show with Nancy at her house in 1964. Since then, I have a love of all forms of music. My high school history teacher introduced me to the classics: Beethoven, Bach, Stravinsky, etcetera. I would go into the library at school, put on headsets and listen to classical music while I studied.

My uncles, for the most part, fought in World War II. Uncle George was a participant in D-Day, and he would tell me stories of fighting Nazis in the hedgerows of Normandy, as a Sgt. He would be given a field promotion to Captain for bravery and saving several comrades. He was a decorated hero and was wounded several times, leaving him with a limp he carried throughout his life. He was awarded the Presidential Unit award and several Purple Hearts. Aside from my parents, he was the most influential person in my life.

My Uncle Bus, Army, would be a participant in the liberation of the Philippine Islands after extensive service in the Pacific.

My Uncle Fred, my namesake, was a decorated Marine. He was a tall stern fellow and was the kindest soul you could ever meet.

My Father was SSgt. in the Army Air Corps stationed in Guam during the Korean War, strategically supporting the war from that tiny island.

One could say service to our country was a family tradition. I had occasions to speak with my Great Grandmother on my father's side about her father, who fought in the Civil War for the North. I did not get much information about him as I was very young at the time.

Never very athletic, I tried out for Little League baseball and didn't make the team. I knew then athletics wasn't for me. In my later years at 15 and 16 I played Junior League baseball sponsored by the American Legion and Vicky's Diner.

I was always a scout, a cub scout, and then a Boy Scout, eventually becoming an Eagle Scout with a silver palm. I also earned the Catholic Boy Scout religious award presented by Francis Cardinal Spellman in Saint Patrick's Cathedral, New York City. I was inducted into Scouting's "Order of the Arrow". My father became very active as a committee member. He eventually became a scoutmaster, and the kids respectfully nicknamed him Kaiser Cadden. As I mentioned, my father was strict and always kept the boys in check. Cub scouts, every Memorial Day (formerly Flag Day), we would March in Hyde Park, NY, and end up at the Hyde Park town hall where Eleanor Roosevelt would speak. I had the privilege as a young boy to see her in person and was present to see her funeral procession, which included the Kennedys, Nikita Khrushchev, and Charles de Gaulle among other world leaders and dignitaries. This would later inspire me to serve my country by joining the Air Force and serving in Vietnam.

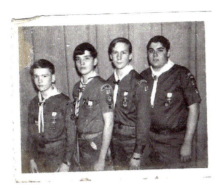

Fred Catholic Award

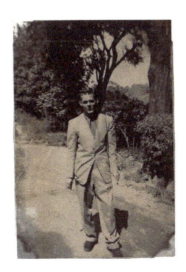

Dad Creek Road

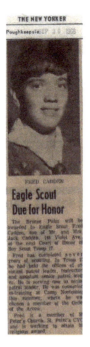

Although I wasn't athletic, I played freshman and junior varsity football, in which I mainly played on the bench. The only time the coach would put me in was if we were winning 40 to nothing, and that happened once against Beacon High School. I was the smallest kid on the team, and I played the position of guard. My number was 69.

I obtained my driver's license when I was 17 and took my girlfriend to the Drive-In the first day, which was a Saturday. I couldn't tell you what the movie was that played. We made love the whole time. She was a gorgeous blonde whom I met when I worked in Food Service at a local hospital. We would deliver patients' food to the floors. I would push the food cart and she would deliver the trays. On the way to the floors, we would stop the elevator in between floors and make out. I know it was not the brightest thing to do, but I was young, dumb, and full of cum. The next morning the family got in the car to head for church. My Mother found a blonde hair that was stuck in the door handle. She immediately turned to my father and said "Jack, what is this blonde hair in the door handle?" They both laughed and turned to look at me as I was cowering in the back seat.

I graduated High School in June of 1969 from Franklin Delano Roosevelt High School in Hyde Park, NY. That summer, after graduation, my buddies and I had the choice of either going to Woodstock or to the boardwalk in Atlantic City, where my friend Chuck wanted to see Busty Russell and her fabulous 50s. Unfortunately, it was decided amongst the five of us that we would go to Atlantic City, and we missed out on the Woodstock music festival, which was the event of a lifetime.

The summer of '69, before starting Junior College, I worked for a local florist delivering flowers and working in the greenhouses, disbudding carnations and scraping and painting the frames on scaffolds with my radio listening to the Miracle Mets. That was the year The Jets won Super Bowl III and the Knicks won the NBA Championship 1969-1970 Season.

The first few semesters of Junior College were Life changing. My friends and I would go to Frank's Bar and Grill which was across the street from the entrance to Marist College. We would pick up girls at Frank's And either go back to a friend's dorm room or go parking. Sometimes when there was only a girl or two in the Bar, My friend Paul and I would play the bowling machine to see who would be the first to approach the prettiest girl and get lucky.

During my third semester, I met a student nurse, Chris. After going to the bar, we would pull in to my boss' driveway in between the greenhouses and park and make love. We dated for several months, and one day, I was in the library studying for my finals when I decided to take a break and call Chris. This was before cell phones, so I called her at her dorm. I asked for Chris and her friend came to the phone and told me that she was in the hospital. She had a miscarriage. I immediately went to be by her side and stayed with her, missing my finals. The best part of valor and responsibility, I asked her to marry me. We sealed the deal at a local Italian restaurant over veal cutlets and a fine chianti.

After flunking my semester, my options were limited. I still had no idea of a major if I continued school, and I did not want to work in a factory. I knew how hard it was on my father, who worked the night shift at Western Publishing, where he eventually became head of the Bookbinder's Union.

Unbeknownst to my parents and everyone else, I went to the Air Force Recruiter in January 1971 and enlisted. I had a high number in the Draft Lottery, so I knew I wasn't going to be drafted into the Army. I felt life expectancy would be higher in the Air Force, and besides, my father served in the Army Air Corp. in Guam leading up to the Korean War.

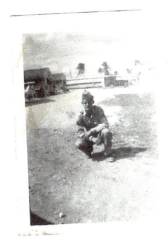 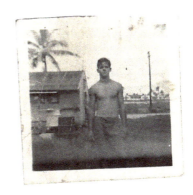

Shirtless Dad in Guam

I grew up in Hyde Park, NY, in the shadow of FDR, so I felt a high sense of duty to serve my country.

My parents didn't say much, but I know it worried my mother. I had a relative Warrant Officer who was shot down in Vietnam and came home an injured War Hero. I had another relative Army Infantry in Vietnam who was wounded and received the Purple Heart. I figured that chances were that I wouldn't even be sent to Vietnam.

I remember my father driving me to the Bus station where I was heading to Albany, the State Capital, to be sworn in, having passed my physical a week earlier. It was the closest I had ever been to my old man. I could see the pride in his eyes and me holding back tears.

In Albany, I took the following oath:

"I, Frederick Leonard Cadden, do hereby acknowledge to have voluntarily enlisted under the conditions prescribed by law, this 25th of February 1971, in the United States Air Force for a period of FOUR (4) years unless sooner discharged by proper authority; and I do solemnly swear (or affirm) that I will support and defend the Constitution of the United States against all enemies, foreign and domestic; that I will bear true faith and allegiance to the same; and that I will obey the orders of the President of the United States and the officers appointed over me, according to regulations, and the Uniform Code of Military Justice, So help me God."

From Albany, I would go to Lackland Air Force Base in San Antonio, Texas, for basic training as my father had done years before when he joined The Army Air Corps.

Basic training was a lot of classrooms, a lot of conditioning and survival training. We were tested extensively to see where Uncle Sam wanted to place us in his Air Force. I enlisted in computer programming, but my scores were not high enough. I was testing next to a guy who had an associate degree in computer programming, and he did not make the grade.

After running my security background check I found out I was going to Medic school and then to Medical Administration Tech school at Shepard Air Force Base in Wichita Falls, Texas. I was an Eagle Scout and had 2 years of Junior College; I am sure that figured somehow into the equation.

Tech School had a lot of work and studying. Our flight group consisted of a cool bunch of guys. We could joke around with each other without fear of racial and social boundaries. The way it should be. Our Staff Sergeant took us to a sleazy bar that had prostitutes. Some had scars on their faces where their pimp or Johns had slashed them with a knife or beer glass. I did not partake, and I think everyone passed on those lovely ladies of the night. While in Tech school, we were given a questionnaire asking about our preferences of where we would like to serve. I put down Worldwide Duty. That is when I got the orders for Vietnam. Not long after, I received a Dear John Letter from Chris. She was breaking off our engagement. Her brother served in the Army in Vietnam, and he was against his sister being engaged while I was over there.

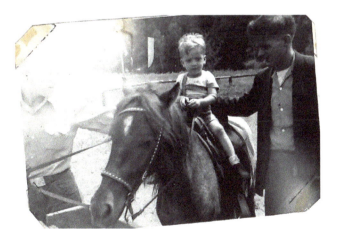

First Pony Ride

"Off to The English Civil War"

Tell me not, sweet; I am unkind.

That from the nunnery

Of thy chaste breast and quiet mind

To warlike arms, I fly.

True, a new mistress now I serve.

The first foe in the field

And with sterner faith, embrace

The sword, a horse, a shield.

Yet this inconsistency is such.

As thou too shalt adore.

I could not love thee, dear, so much

Loved I not honor more.

Richard Lovelace (1618-1657)

After getting this wonderful news, I proceeded to absorb a 6-pack of Colt 45 Malt Liqueur tall boys.

This rendered me incapable of acting in a logical manner. I decided that I would go AWOL and fly back to New York and set things right. I packed my bag and told my roommate of my plans and left. I made it as far as the base front gate and passed out under the flag poles. That is where I woke up the next morning. I gathered myself and my AWOL Bag and went back to my barracks and my room. The fact that I remained untouched the night before led me to believe that my roommate notified our SSgt. And the base command decided to let me stay there unapproached. My roommate and I never spoke about it, and nothing was ever mentioned during the remainder of my stay at Tech School.

After this incident, I called the Nursing school Dorm and asked for my ex-fiancé; her roommate told me that Chris had met a guy, became pregnant and had a miscarriage and that the guy had fled to California. I then learned that Chris was in a psychiatric institution.

After graduation from Tech School, our Tech Sargeant told us that some of us would go to Vietnam, Republic of. I learned of my assignment. I had a 30-day leave, and I first went to visit Chris' Grandmother, who told me which institution she was in. I went to visit her, and they would only allow me to visit her in a separate padded room. I learned she had to be restrained during the visit. My visit was brief, and I was saddened and began to pray for her. Since then, she would only write to me after she had a nervous breakdown.

I always wrote her back until my last visit after leaving the Air Force. I brought her a Scottish puppet I purchased at a shop in Cambridge, England. She was Scottish and loved puppets. I never heard from her again.

Of my 30-day leave, I spent a week with my parents and the rest with my friends partying hardy before my deployment to Vietnam.

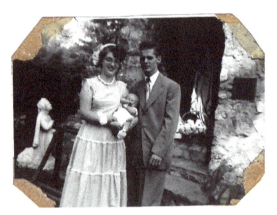

Fred Christening

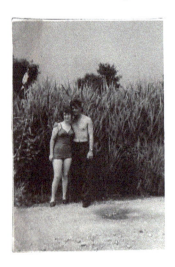

Mom and Dad

Chapter II
Cam Ranh Bay, Republic of Vietnam 1971 – 1972

I flew out of Albany, NY, enroute to Tacoma, Washington, where I would spend overnight in a motel and embark the next morning on a Flying Tiger's transport to Cam Ranh Bay, where I was assigned to the 483rd US Air Force Hospital as a member of the US Air Force Medical Corps.

It was about 7:30 PM when I arrived at the Medic Squadron Area. I was told to stow my gear and report to the Squadron Headquarters area, where I was told "Training films" were being shown and it was mandatory that I attend. As I approached the area, I saw a projection on one of the concrete revetments that all the guys in my Squadron were gathered around and attentively watching. They were Blue Movies, nowadays commonly known as Porn. Not being shy, I sat down and joined in my training. That was my first night in Vietnam. After the training, I wanted to shower; after being in flight all those hours I could gag a maggot. As I entered the Latrine area and headed toward the shower, there were four naked Vietnamese women or girls leaving and wrapping towels around their firm young bodies. I thought to myself, hmmmm, I wouldn't mind sharing a shower with those beauties. They were sic-lo girls or prostitutes that were allowed on base each evening. As I would later learn, you had to be careful because you didn't know which ones were Viet Cong that were conveniently placed on base. Cam Ranh Bay Air Base was built on a huge Sand Dune. The sand was everywhere and in everything. One had to wear flip-flops or shoes when traveling the few yards from the Hootch area to the Latrine because some of the VC girls would pee on razor blades and stick them in the sand for the purpose of injuring and infecting us medics. Medics are always the first to be targeted to crush morale and prevent the healing of the wounded.

My job was to man the Hospital Command Post during the evening shift 7 at night till 7 AM. I worked 2 on and 2 off. If an aircraft came back to base on a wing and a prayer from sorties, I would dispatch ambulances to the flight line and notify all medical personnel. The same was true when the base was under attack.

I was also responsible for the processing of reports for all Deaths, seriously ill, and very seriously ill. I processed patients for Aeromedical Evacuation moving sick and wounded through the 26th Aeromedical Staging Facility.

See Job description and Performance Report.

FACTS AND SPECIFIC ACHIEVEMENTS: A1C Cadden has performed his duties as Night Admissions and Dispositions Clerk with efficiency and enthusiasm. As Night Admissions and Dispositions Clerk, Airman Cadden had to perform his duties without supervision. Since the Hospital Command Post was located in the Admission and Disposition Office, part of Airman Cadden's duties was to monitor the radios in case of an emergency. In case of emergency, it was necessary for him to recall all key personnel and assist in coordinating any medical operations required under the situation. On many occasions, he performed these duties alone until assistance arrived. He always handled these duties with the utmost competency. A1C Cadden also had to initiate and process the reports for all deaths, seriously ill, and very seriously ill and several patient status reports. These reports were always done in a very neat and competent manner. A1C Cadden's attention to the many details involved in the administrative processing of patients for aeromedical evacuation has been a significant factor in the smooth, expedient flow of sick and wounded personnel through the 26th Aeromedical Staging Facility. **STRENGTHS:** A1C Cadden's maturity and adaptability to the different situation encountered in his daily duties has been a great asset to his job performance as well as to himself. As a first term airman, A1C Cadden has shown an ability to take the initiative. He performs his duties very enthusiastically and at present time is performing the duties of a sergeant. **EDUCATIONAL AND TRAINING ACCOMPLISHMENTS:** At present time A1C Cadden is involved in OJT training for his five level. **SUGGESTED ASSIGNMENTS:** A1C Cadden has performed very competently as Admissh n and disposition clerk; however, he should be given the opportunity to work in other areas of his career field such as the Business Office, Registrar Office or the Administrative Services. **OTHER COMMENTS:** All duties during this reporting period were performed in Southeast Asia.

Ronald Elder
RONALD ELDER, SGT
483rd USAF HOSPITAL (PACAF)

ADDITIONAL INDORSEMENT: I have observed A1C Cadden's duty performance on a daily basis during this report period. I have found him to be a most dependable young airman with exceptional growth potential. I concur with this report as rendered.

Robert L. Casey
ROBERT L. CASEY, MSGT
483rd USAF HOSPITAL (PACAF)

ADDITIONAL INDORSEMENT: I concur with the reporting and indorsing official. A1C Cadden has performed his duties in an exceptional manner. He has proven to be a very capable member of the administrative section of this hospital.

Earl W. Plaugher
EARL W. PLAUGHER, Major, 483rd USAF Hosp, PACAF, Administrator, 20 April 1972

One morning, as I was being relieved of my night duties, I was walking back to my hootch, and I noticed a crowd gathering next door. Security police were all over. I thought to myself, did they find my stash? Lol. Turns out, there happened to be a VC Major living next door as a prostitute, and they caught her with a transmitter and receiver. Her mission was to plot the location of us Medics and attack us. She could have slashed our throats at any time. There were several other attempts of Viet Cong infiltrators sneaking on base sent to plot Medics location. I heard they were interrogated, although I discovered nothing about their fate.

As a base, we were rocketed every other night, it seemed. Luckily for us, half the Russian and Chinese rockets were duds and they just stuck in the sand without exploding. Kept our ordinance guys busy.

After a month of being in the country, Sappers infiltrated our base and blew up our Ammo Dump on 25 August 1971. My buddy, Steve and I were having a cigarette break outside of the Emergency Room and talking to an Army Master Sergeant who had just come in from the Bush. As we were talking, we saw a flash that lit up the sky as bright as daylight, then the largest boom I had experienced up until that point. We were looking around and could not see the Master Sergeant. After the flash, he jumped behind the 3-foot brick wall that circled the perimeter of the hospital. Needless to say, we quickly joined him. There were clusters of 5/500 lb. bombs going off all night. I later learned from documents about the attack, declassified in the 1980's, there were barrels of Napalm, and I assumed Agent Orange. Agent Orange (which was not officially mentioned in the report) was in the mix that we were breathing for weeks. The report also stated that the attack was the most devastating and costly of the entire war, with over $10.9 Million munitions damaged in 1971 money.

OEClASSIFIEO BY AF/HOH IAW f.0.12958 tHlfNDfD) OH£, 20080718

APPROVED   FOR PUBLIC RHEAS£

PROJECT CHECO SOUTHEAST ASIA REPORT

ATTACK ON CAM RANN

25 AUGUST 1971

SPECIAL RIPORT

UNCLASSIFIED

DEPARTMENT OF THE AIR FORCE
HEADQUARTERS PACIFIC AIR FORCES
APO SAN FRANCISCO 96553

PROJECT CHECO REPORTS

The counterinsurgency and unconventional warfare environment of Southeast Asia has resulted in the employment of USAF airpower to meet a multitude of requirements. The varied applications of airpower have involved the full spectrum of USAF aerospace vehicles, support equipment, and manpower. As a result, there has been an accumulation of operational data and experiences that, as a priority, must be collected, documented, and analyzed as to current and future impact upon USAF policies, concepts, and doctrine.

Fortunately, the value of collecting and documenting our SEA experiences was recognized at an early date. In 1962, Hq USAF directed CINCPACAF to establish an activity that would be primarily responsive to Air Staff requirements and direction, and would provide timely and analytical studies of USAF combat operations in SEA.

Project CHECO, an acronym for Contemporary Historical Examination of Current Operations, was established to meet this Air Staff requirement. Managed by Hq PACAF, with elements at Hq 7AF and 7AF/13AF, Project CHECO provides a scholarly, "on-going" historical examination, documentation, and reporting on USAF policies, concepts, and doctrine in PACOM. This CHECO report is part of the overall documentation and examination which is being accomplished. It is an authentic source for an assessment of the effectiveness of USAF airpower in PACOM when used in proper context. The reader must view the study in relation to the events and circumstances at the time of its preparation--recognizing that it was prepared on a contemporary basis which restricted perspective and that the author's research was limited to records available within his local headquarters area.

ERNEST C. HARDIN, JR., Major General, USAF
Chief of Staff

DEPARTMENT OF THE AIR FORCE
HEADQUARTERS PACIFIC AIR FORCES
APO SAN FRANCISCO 96553

DOAD   15 December 1971

Project CHECO Report, "Attack on Cam Ranh, 25 Aug 71" (U)

SEE DISTRIBUTION PAGE

1. Attached is a SECRET NOFORN document. It shall be transported, stored, safeguarded, and accounted for in accordance with applicable security directives. SPECIAL HANDLING REQUIRED, NOT RELEASABLE TO FOREIGN NATIONALS. The information contained in this document will not be disclosed to foreign nations or their representatives. Retain or destroy in accordance with AFR 205-1. Do not return.

2. This letter does not contain classified information and may be declassified if attachment is removed from it.

FOR THE COMMANDER IN CHIEF

ROBERT E. HILLER   1 Atch
Director of Operations Analysis   Proj CHECO Rprt (S/NF),
DCS/Operations   15 Dec 71

iii

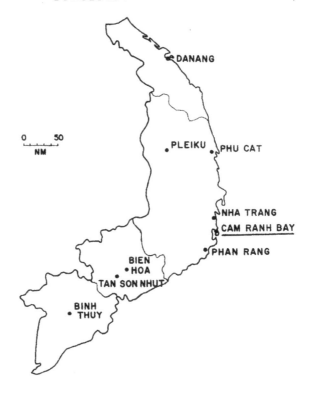

Map of Republic of Vietnam showing location of Cam Ranh Bay Air Base.

FIGURE 1

INTRODUCTION

During the early morning hours of 25 August 1971, the Tri-Service Ammunition Storage Area (TSASA) of Cam Ranh Bay Air Base (CRBAB) was the target of a highly destructive sapper attack. Bright fireballs illuminated the sky and shock waves travelled for miles around, awakening a sleeping population. By hitting what the populace perceived to be a "well-defended" target at an opportune time, the Viet Cong achieved a desired propaganda effect four days prior to the national elections. The sappers penetrated the munitions storage area, attached time-delayed explosive charges to its contents, and fled unharmed. In coordination with the intrusion, hostile forces fired two volleys of rockets onto the other side of the base, apparently to divert the attention of security personnel.

Massive detonations lasted for several hours and scattered live munitions over a wide area. The success of the attack can be measured by the extent of damage. Approximately six thousand tons of ammunition, valued in excess of $10.3 million, were destroyed. The explosions caused $174,000 damage to the TSASA, and the concussion effects alone resulted in $99,000 damage to real estate on the base proper.[1] Fortunately, there were no fatalities; five security policemen received minor wounds.[2]

This report describes the conditions that prevailed prior to the attack, the attack itself, and the subsequent defensive changes. A description of the Cam Ranh Special Sector (CRSS) and, specifically, the TSASA, the forewarnings of the attack, and a chronology of the assault are followed by an analysis. The analysis focuses on the vulnerabilities and deficiencies of base defense and precedes the account of resultant changes in security measures. The conclusion alludes to the lessons learned for planning of security operations in the future.

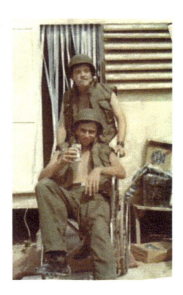

My Buddy Daryl and myself, the morning after the attack

I am still suffering from the effects of that night due to exposure to Toxins that we were exposed to. The VA has awarded me 100 % service-connected Disability. I have no feeling in my legs from my feet to mid-thigh, Neuropathy and Diabetes.

The VC finally did succeed in killing some Medics. Cam Ranh Bay was home to not only the Air Force, but also Army and Naval Bases. VC had attacked the Army Medics, tossing satchel charges as they skipped through the barracks. I stuffed body bags, and we loaded them in the cooler for Graves Registration. There was one casualty that I kept seeing. The patient had his chest blown open, and we were frantically applying suction so the Chief Surgeon could do his work. He was saying, "Oh My God, Oh My God" repeatedly. I can never forget that. We evacuated him to Clarke Air Base in the Philippines, and I later learned he died enroute. Years later, I visited the Philippines and the medical facility at Clarke in an effort to pray and put my demons to rest. It did not work. As Joseph Galloway, Journalist and Reporter, famously said, "Once you see War, you always see it." No truer words have ever been spoken.

Now, as I thought I was somewhat educated and at 20, I thought I knew all there was to know about the world, I was in for a very rude awakening. A Buddy of mine was being reassigned back to the States. Before he left, he asked me if I would be interested in taking over his class. It would be teaching English to Vietnamese Civilians who worked on the base. Being a History/English major, I said yes and then started off on my brief Teaching Career.

Teaching English to the Vietnamese Civilians who worked on base was a rewarding experience because I learned about the people, their customs, and their country. It was a welcome break from the traumas of war. I got to know each student, whose ages ranged from 17 – 50. They had a basic knowledge of English but needed grammar and pronunciation skills. It was sad when they ended the program in preparation for the base eventually closing. I received a citation of gratitude from the Vietnamese Government which was placed in my Service Record. Looking back, I wondered whatever happened to my students as their duties on base ended and they were sent back to their homes.

I remember Christmas 1971. Christmas was always a very special time for me. Being away from home on the opposite side of the world from my family in a War Zone was painful for me. I spent the day in my hootch during a monsoon downpour with a bottle of Vodka listening to Rolling Stones' Sticky Fingers, Jethro Tull's Aqualung, The Who's Who's Next. We were preparing for another TET Offensive, filling sandbags and watching our tracer rounds going off periodically through the night. The Offensive never occurred.

President Nixon, our Commander-in-Chief, decided to implement an amnesty program for Drug Abusers. Those soldiers whose urine tested positive for opiates were entered into our facility before being sent home. It didn't take long for dudes in the bush to figure out that all they needed was to take enough heroine that would barely turn their drug test positive. Some actually took drugs thinking they could pass much of the time sleeping through the war. Our wards were filled with GI's.

After a short period of time, they would move us closer to the hospital as Airmen were reassigned to other hospitals in Southeast Asia or to the States. As time passed, we were eventually housed in a hospital ward fashioned into a barracks-type situation. The Hospital chow hall was closed, and we ate c-rations for the duration. The close quarters in that ward had seen a few guys lose it and had to be subdued and eventually sent home.

Taking that Freedom Bird Home was rewarding and gave me a great feeling of relief. I Survived "The Nam!!!!"

We had a brief layover in Tokyo and then on to San Francisco. Still in uniform, Dress Blues, I purchased my ticket to Albany, NY.

Reaching Albany, I quickly changed into my civies as I did not know what to expect on my arrival back home. I took the train from Albany to Poughkeepsie and called my Father to pick me up at the terminal. He told me not to tell my mother so we could surprise her at her place of work. She was so ecstatic. It was a wonderful welcome home.

Looking back, I was torn with emotions and wanted to put it all behind me and not think or mention Vietnam ever again. Well, decades passed, and I felt like I had to put my experience to writing and celebrate the fact that I am a proud Vietnam Veteran.

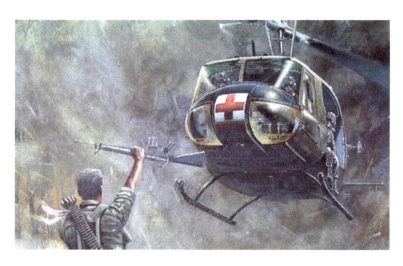

A Veteran's Day Reflection (2016)

THE THINGS WE BEAT OURSELVES UP FOR DAY TO DAY THAT WE MUST RISE ABOVE AND PUT INTO PERSPECTIVE BECAUSE OF OUR EXPERIENCES OVER THERE. THERE IS NOT A DAY THAT GOES BY THAT I DON'T WONDER WHY ME? AFTER WITNESSING SO MANY SUFFER AND LOSE LIMB AND LIFE, MANY OF US ASK, WHY DID I ESCAPE UNSCATHED AFTER DECADES OF DENIAL AND SELF-BLAME? I CAN PROUDLY TURN AROUND AND SAY IT WAS BECAUSE I WAS MEANT TO BE THERE FOR THEM, AND THEN I BECOME THANKFUL.

Fred Cadden – Life Member VFW Post 4228 Titusville, FL

USAF Medical Corps.

26th Aeromedical Staging Facility

Cam Ranh Bay, Republic of Vietnam 1971-1972

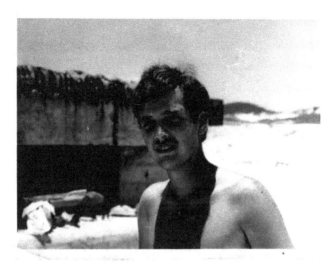

Me at the beach in Cam Ranh Bay Next to a Japanese Pill Box from WW II

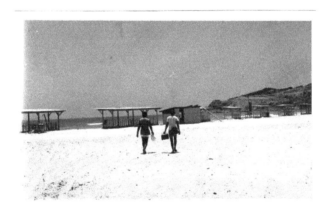

Above is a photo of Cam Ranh Bay Beach. It was soothing and refreshing to get away for just a little while amidst the chaos and turmoil of the war. These are 2 of my buddies, one a male nurse and the other an Operating Room Tech.

To feel the warmth and cadence of the waves crashing on the beach, reminded me of the vastness and power of God's work. I knew that one day I would leave this place and that the good and the bad days would haunt me for the rest of my days.

As we walked the beach there were staunch reminders of the war. We would come across makeshift mortar tubes made of bamboo left by the Viet Cong. One day, as we were returning to the base, I came across a live round from a grenade launcher. I brought it to the guard on duty, and he shouted, "Stop!! Don't move and put the round slowly on the ground and step away; that is a 40 mm Grenade". He then called a demolition crew to come out. By this time, I didn't know whether to shit or fly…...

The Demolition guy finally came and just casually walked up, put it in his back pocket, said, "Nothing to worry about," and walked back to the base. Evidently, one of our guys had lost it on patrol. Below is a cash of 40 mm grenades, the most powerful grenade used in grenade launchers in the war. I was relieved, to say the least.

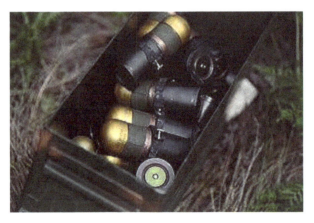

Chapter III
England: 10th Tactical Reconnaissance Wing RAF Alconbury 1972-1975

After Serving in Vietnam, you were offered the assignment of your choice. I chose Europe.

I was told that my next assignment would be at Torrejon Air Base in Madrid, Spain. I was so excited to get this choice assignment. Spanish Senoritas, I am here to relieve you of your virginity! . My excitement was short-lived, however, when my orders were changed to RAF Alconbury in the UK. I was still in Europe, and the locals spoke my language. I was happy with the choice the Air Force made. It turns out that the Airman I would be replacing was caught with drugs and was awaiting to be sent back to the States.

At home, as a youth, I watched "The World at War" Series on PBS and I was fascinated with The Royal Air Force and its role in World War II. Now, I would technically be a contributing part of the RAF and NATO for the next three years.

From the Vietnam War to the Cold War. It was a privilege to serve and be a part of history.

Our Mission was to run reconnaissance over Eastern Europe. Our planes were equipped with sophisticated, state-of-the-art cameras. There was a US Army detachment on base that would interpret the photos captured by the cameras.

I would be the sergeant in charge of Registrar Services at the 10th TAC Hospital. My duties were to oversee Medical Records and patient appointments, and coordinate with staff doctors, The Lab, the Pharmacy, and Flight Surgeons Office. I would complete and distribute daily reports for the hospital.

We were just a 10-bed hospital that would eventually downsize to 2 beds, and then finally, we just became an outpatient clinic. Patients would be referred to the large hospital at RAF Lakenheath, just several miles away, when required.

The base is located just outside of Cambridge, England, in Huntingdon. It is still operated by the US as the 501st Combat Support Wing.

Settling In

I flew commercially into Heathrow Airport in London. A bus greeted us bound for RAF Alconbury and RAF Lakenheath. I was assigned to my barracks room and began to make myself comfortable. My roommate was Ken, but everyone called him "Mad Dog". Ken was not there at the time, and I made myself at home. I came to find out the moniker of "Mad Dog" did not suit him. We became good friends and had similar interests. Our barracks were evenly integrated, with all kinds of music filling the hallway.

The Airman I was replacing lived off base and was relieved of duty. I met him later as he was a friend of my roommate. I reported initially to the Staff Sergeant running the Registrar's Office. He taught me the job, and after, he and his wife were transferred back to the United States.

I became friends with all the guys in my Squadron, and we would go to the Airman's club and pick up dates (girls that were bussed in from surrounding environs). It was fun, and we spent many late weekends dancing and stumbling back to the barracks. One of my roommates and a good friend, was Michael. We had two bedrooms separated by a door that we kept open at all times. Now Michael was black and was known for his rather large manhood and would do what he called were sex exercises. One Saturday night as I was sleeping, I heard A loud yell and a woman shouting to her friend, "my God, look at the size of that thing"!!

We would go on jaunts to London and see all the sights, Changing of the Guard, National Museum, Piccadilly, Soho.

I enjoyed the British culture and would venture to pubs and restaurants around Cambridge. I met an Irish girl who had a 2-year-old little girl that was as cute as a button. I was smitten by both her and her mom, and we were shortly married.

At my bachelor party, my friends from the Medic Squadron and I went to a friend's house, where we roasted a whole pig on a spicket outside. After much drink and food, my friends held me down while my good friend Pete shaved my pubic hair (a Squadron Tradition).

I moved into her apartment, and we became a family. Sadly, the marriage lasted only six months, and then we got an annulment.

After living off base, I did not want to go back to barracks life. I stayed with a friend and his wife In Stilton near Peterborough. Stilton was famous for Stilton Cheese. I would spend many hours exploring Peterborough's Cathedral, making Brass Rubbings of the inscriptions and sarcophagi of deceased Clergy and Royalty.

I was promoted to Sergeant and was a Non-Commissioned Officer in Charge of Registrar Services. There, I oversaw Medical Records, Clinic Appointments, and daily reports of Clinic activities.

Chapter IV
Peaceholme

I met a friend (Ron) who worked in the base Personnel, and I was invited to move in with him and another Airman from my Squadron (Tom) to a village called Needingworth. Across the street was "The Queen's Head," a local Pub. Our house was a renovated 200-year-old Pub with a wine cellar. The Plaque on the front door read "PEACEHOLME".

Wales; Memorial Day Weekend

After a few months, Ron, myself and another friend, Mike, decided to go camping in Wales for the Memorial Day Weekend. We found a campground that accommodated tents, and you could rent a small trailer onsite. After being there a day, we met 2 Canadian girls who rented a trailer next to our camp. We invited the girls to our tent, and we were drinking, singing, and having a good time. After a while, the girls said good night and went back to their trailer. After an hour it started to pour down rain, soaking the tent and leaking on one side. I made the command decision to give up my side of the tent and headed straight for the girls' trailer. Once inside, I began to dry off, and the girls removed my clothes, and we each had a satisfying night. My poor buddies in the tent refused to talk to me on the way back to Needingworth.

There is a small grocery store next to Peaceholme that was owned by our landlord's sister, Ann. As we arrived home, there was a note on our door from Ann saying, "Don't go in; come and see me first." Ron and I did not know what to make of it, so we went to Ann's. Evidently, Tom took some hallucinogens and started a fire in the kitchen with coal from the fireplace. When Police and Fire arrived there, he was raving about burning the Fascists. He was arrested and carted off to jail. We never heard from him again, as arson is a Capital Offence in Great Britain. I can only assume he was eventually handed over to US Authorities and incarcerated in the States.

Everywhere there was soot and ash. The Landlord was good about cleaning it up and repainting.

We lived in it for several weeks.

European Road Trip

Ron's friend TK from Detroit, a Civilian with long hair and a beard, came to stay.

Ron had recently purchased a brand-new MG Midget. The three of us decided to take a road trip. We took a ferry from Dover to Calais. Down through France to Paris, visited the Notre Dame Cathedral. We travelled through the countryside to Bordeau. Driving through the Pyrenees into Spain was quite an adventure. At times, the road narrowed to merely a cow or donkey path. The MG Midget did well, with yours truly stuffed into the back.

In Spain, we drove to Zaragosa, where we stopped and rested. People all along the way were friendly and pleased to help us. Driving down the Costa Del Sol, we stopped at Barcelona where we found friendly accommodation and great food. Eating Paella at a restaurant on the beach, we met a German couple on vacation, and we sat around drinking wine and sharing stories.

Reaching the South of Spain, we took a Ferry from Gibraltar to Ceuta. We attempted to enter Morocco, but officials would not let us in thinking TK was a Hippie with his long hair and beard. Ron and I had no problems with our Military I.D. and military haircuts. We turned around and went back to Spain, however.

We drove straight through to Amsterdam where we spent the night in the Hans Brinker Youth Hostel. I had to head back to base the next day as I only had two weeks' leave. The ride back to England was an experience I will never forget. It was late September and bitter cold onboard the Hover Craft. It was a bumpy and cold ride. The only thing I had to keep me warm was a Sarape that I purchased in Spain.

The British Experience

The three of us became good friends. On his trip to Needingworth, TK met some friends along the way. All were British Nationals, and it was the 70s! Most had an association with Kings College Cambridge, either students or friends of students. We would go visit them, or they would visit us.

We had one friend who streaked the Queen's Head Pub one night. It turned out to be a form of advertisement for the Pub. The most exciting thing to happen to that sleepy little town in years. You could hear the Pub Patrons say, "Must be Those Crazy Yanks across the street". The next morning, the Pub had posters up: "Come to the Queen's Head where Streakers roam the night."

On one trip to a Pub in London a bunch of friends and I drove back with a young English lady, and we all ended up in the living room listening to music until 3 A.M. in the morning. As I noticed the young lady dozing off, I offered her to go upstairs, and she could stay in my bedroom. After about 15 minutes I bid my mates good night and went upstairs to find a naked young lady in my bed. What would a young red blooded American Airman do in this situation? I removed my clothes and jumped in bed. Immediately she "grasped the root of my existence"!!! We made love the rest of the morning. She was amazing.

As I mentioned earlier, there was a detachment of Army Personnel at RAF Alconbury who conducted photo interpretations of our reconnaissance photos. There was a blond WAC named Zoey attached to the unit that everyone on base tried to get to know. One day Ron had asked Zoey to join us at a Pub close to the base. We were all at the Pub drinking our pints of bitter when Zoey came over to me and said, "I would rather be with you! What are you going to do about It?" Well, I almost dropped my beer and was so surprised that this chick, who everyone on base wanted to be with, would want to be with me. I moved in with her and her 3-year-old daughter. This lasted for six months.

After a while, Ron was discharged, and he and TK left for another trek across Europe. I still visited our English friends at

Kings College, who seemed to think that I had walked out of an F. Scott Fitzgerald novel. One of my friends was the son of the Pakistani Ambassador to Great Britain. He had a fancy for Southern Comfort, and I would occasionally bring him a bottle from the base exchange. One day after finals, he got so wasted on Southern Comfort that it was hysterical.

- Still smitten with the travelling bug, I drove to Scotland for New Year's Eve. There, at a Hotel and pub in Sterling, the clock struck midnight, and the most beautiful Scottish Damsel came up and kissed me on the cheek. I returned the favor, and we spent the rest of the night together making love.
- One of our friends was from Hastings. I was excited to go there because I learned about the Battle of Hastings 1066 in High School between the Norman-French Army of William the Duke of Normandy and the Anglo-Saxon King Harold Godwinson. William defeated Harold and killed the Anglo-Saxon King. It was an unexpected trip and one I thoroughly enjoyed.
- Next was Stone Henge in Wiltshire. A fascinating structure that I had always read about and was fascinated with the Druids and legends of how it was built by Merlin the Magician who levitated the blocks in position obtained from a site in Wales many miles away.

- I visited Canterbury Cathedral and saw the final resting place of Thomas Becket. I always wanted to see the Cathedral ever since I saw the Movie "Becket" with Richard Burton.

On to Stratford -on-Avon where I saw Shakespear's home. Visiting the Globe Theater, I became friends with stagehands during a dress rehearsal of Hamlet. They invited me back to their apartment, and we drank wine and talked about life. I love England!

On occasion, it was necessary for me to camp overnight during my travels. One night, I camped in a farmer's field and was reading a book by Kurt Vonnegut; I believe it was "Breakfast of Champions". I came to the part where an alien crash-landed in a farmer's field and the alien went to the farmhouse for help. It so happened that the only form of communication the alien had was by Farting and Tap Dancing. The farmer grabbed his shotgun and blew away the alien. Somewhere in a farmer's field in England, in the middle of the night, you could hear me laughing hysterically.

Love at the Clinic

I worked with this beautiful and amazing woman who I fell in love with. We would go on dates where we would come to Peaceholme and listen to "The Best of the Byrds" and Bob Dylan. We went to see Blazing Saddles at a theater in Cambridge. She was black, and this was the 70's. Interracial relationships were somewhat acceptable in England.

Our relationship was purely platonic, but we had a connection that ran deep within our souls.

On our last date, I dropped her off at her barracks, we kissed, and then she said we could not continue because it would never be accepted back home. She was from Detroit. Her parents moved there when she was a child after the KKK burned a cross on the family's lawn in Mississippi. After I came home from England, I called her barracks several times, but she refused to take my calls. I love her to this day.

The Circumcision

One of the doctors who removed a pesky cyst on my arm offered to do my circumcision. I agreed, and we scheduled the operation. My friend assisted, and after the operation, I was groggy, and he brought me to a mutual friend's house. After being there for about 20 minutes, our friend started playing blue movies (Porn). That was a cruel joke, and I was popping Amyl Nitrate capsules the whole visit to keep me from busting my stitches.

After moving to Houston, I saw a PBS special on Micro-Surgery, and it featured the doctor who performed my circumcision. He was a pioneer in Micro-Surgery. That is not to have anything to do with the size of my manhood.

Bon Voyage

It was finally time for me to leave Jolly Old England and start my journey home, and on to Houston. My friends at Kings College Cambridge gave me a huge send-off, along with some of my co-workers. It was a party in the basement of King's College where my good friend had a band, and they were playing all night with my friend Eddie Bo from the clinic blowing the saxophone!

I will never forget my experiences there and all the people I befriended and came to love.

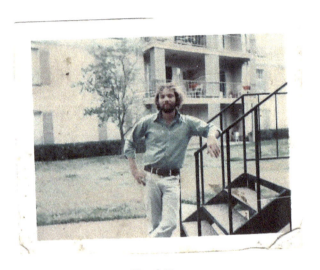

Fred Houston

Chapter V
Houston, Texas – The Early Years

Arrival in Houston: A City of Opportunity

The spring of 1975 marked the beginning of a new chapter in my life as I arrived in Houston, Texas. The city was undergoing a transformation fueled by the oil boom, and it was an exciting time to be there. The contrast between Houston's humid, warm April air and the cool, sometimes harsh British climate was striking. Houston's climate, though sweltering, was a symbol of the city's burgeoning prosperity, driven by its role as the Oil Capital of the World. The city seemed to exude an energy that was both exhilarating and overwhelming.

Walking through Houston felt like stepping into a bustling hive of activity. The streets were alive with the sound of construction, the hum of heavy machinery, and the chatter of workers. Everywhere you looked, new developments were springing up. The city's rapid expansion was visible in the way it consumed the surrounding areas, with new subdivisions and housing developments sprouting up at an astonishing rate. It was a city on the move, a place where anything seemed possible if you were willing to work hard and seize the opportunities.

Cable Slabs: Building the Future

My entry into Houston's dynamic environment came through a summer job arranged by my friend Chuck, who had grown up with me in New York. Chuck's father owned a construction company named "Cable Slabs," which was at the forefront of revolutionary building technology. The company specialized in a new method of foundation construction that replaced the traditional re-bar with a system involving steel cables.

Cable Slabs used an innovative technique where engineers would design the layout of the slab and place cables in a crisscross pattern within the trenches. The cables, once stressed to the correct PSI, created a foundation so robust that it was rumored a helicopter could lift it intact without causing any cracks. Although I never witnessed this impressive feat firsthand, the idea of such a strong foundation was a testament to the advanced technology we were working with.

My job at Cable Slabs was physically demanding. I was responsible for stressing the cables to the appropriate PSI and then inserting wedges to lock them in place. The summer heat in Houston was relentless, and the work was grueling. Despite the physical exhaustion, I found a sense of pride in the work and acquired a great tan to boot. The knowledge that I was contributing to the construction of homes and buildings in a city experiencing unprecedented growth was deeply satisfying.

To escape the oppressive heat, my colleagues and I would often seek refuge in a nearby 7/11, standing in front of the refrigeration units to cool off before heading back to the job site. The camaraderie among the workers made the long days more bearable. We shared stories, joked around, and found solace in each other's company.

Houston's Nightlife: A City That Never Sleeps

The Houston of the mid-1970s was not just about work; it was also about play. The city's nightlife was vibrant and unrelenting, reflecting the energy and prosperity of the era. With the influx of oil money, Houston had become a playground for those seeking entertainment, dining, and socializing.

The allure of Houston's nightlife was irresistible. My paychecks, hard-earned from long hours of labor, seemed to vanish as quickly as they were earned. The city offered a wide range of activities, from lively nightclubs to upscale restaurants. Each night was an opportunity to explore a new facet of Houston's social scene, and I found myself swept up in the excitement.

The nightlife wasn't just about indulgence; it was also about forging connections and experiencing life in a city that never seemed to sleep. From dancing to live music to savoring the diverse culinary offerings, Houston's nightlife was a reflection of the city's dynamic spirit. Every evening brought new adventures and new faces, and I relished the chance to immerse myself in the vibrant culture.

The University of Houston: Balancing Education and Work

Recognizing the importance of education, I decided to continue my studies at the University of Houston. My friend Jim and I moved from the west side of the city to the Cougar Apartments, conveniently located just a block from the campus. This proximity was crucial, as navigating Houston's sprawling layout without a vehicle was a challenge.

I enrolled as a History and English Teacher Education major, eager to make the most of the educational opportunities available. However, despite my enthusiasm and dedication, I soon realized that my VA benefits were insufficient to cover all my expenses. The cost of living in Houston, combined with the demands of my coursework, made it clear that I needed to find a job to support myself.

A New Opportunity: Joske's of Houston

During this period, I met Rick in a History of the Theater class. Our shared interest in history and academic pursuits led to a strong friendship. Rick was working part-time in the New Accounts section of Joske's of Houston Credit Department, and when he mentioned an opening, I saw it as an opportunity to both earn money and gain valuable work experience.

The role at Joske's involved running credit reports for individuals applying for credit cards and contract sales, such as TVs and furniture. The work required attention to detail and a strong understanding of financial systems. I quickly adapted to the responsibilities, learning how to handle sensitive information and provide excellent customer service.

The job offered a flexible schedule, allowing me to continue attending classes during the day. It was a demanding role, but the experience was invaluable. I learned about the intricacies of credit systems and developed skills that would serve me well in the future.

The work was rewarding in its own way, providing a sense of stability and contributing to my overall growth.

Weekend Escapes: Galveston and King Neptune

Weekends provided a welcome respite from the demands of work and school. Rick and I would often escape to his parents' beach house in Galveston. The beach house was a sanctuary where we could relax and enjoy the simpler pleasures of life. Our weekends in Galveston were filled with fishing, floundering, and enjoying the fresh seafood that Rick's mother would prepare.

One of our favorite activities was gigging for flounder in the bay. Armed with lanterns and gigs, we ventured into the dark waters, carefully avoiding the stingrays that could be mistaken for flounder. The thrill of the hunt and the camaraderie with friends made these outings unforgettable. We would bring along jugs of rum and fruit punch, adding to the sense of adventure.

One night, after a few drinks, I jokingly declared myself "King Neptune," and the nickname stuck. It became a playful moniker that my friends used to refer to me, a reminder of the fun and camaraderie we shared during those weekends. The beach house became a symbol of friendship and escape, a place where we could let go of our worries and simply enjoy each other's company.

Hermann Hospital: A New Chapter

After several months at Joske's, I decided to apply for a position at Hermann Hospital, the oldest hospital in Houston. The role of Medical Records Supervisor seemed like a perfect fit, given my experience as a Registrar in the Air Force. I was eager to transition into a more stable career and apply the skills I had acquired in the military to a civilian setting.

The hiring process was thorough, but my background as a veteran worked in my favor. I was hired and began working at the hospital, starting with a period of orientation to familiarize myself with the systems and procedures. The transition from retail to healthcare was challenging, but I quickly adapted to the new environment.

Working the night shift came with its own set of responsibilities, including the duty of overseeing the morgue. It was a part of the job that few people saw, but it was essential to the hospital's operations. One night, a worker from the Houston Eye Bank came to collect donated eyes from a recently deceased cancer patient. He invited me to observe the procedure, and I agreed.

The experience was both surreal and educational. When the optic nerve was cut, it made a sound reminiscent of a .22-caliber gunshot. It was a stark reminder of the delicate nature of life and the importance of our work. The role of Medical Records Supervisor was demanding, but it was also deeply fulfilling. It required precision, organization, and a strong sense of responsibility, qualities that I took pride in embodying.

A Supervisor's Challenge: The Great Records Conversion

One of the most significant challenges I faced as a Medical Records Supervisor was the task of converting 35,000 medical records from an alpha filing system to a terminal digit filing system. The project was daunting, and the sheer volume of records was overwhelming. It was a task that required meticulous planning and execution.

The conversion involved reorganizing thousands of records to improve efficiency and accessibility. It was a complex process that demanded attention to detail and a commitment to ensuring that the new system would function smoothly. I worked diligently, often putting in long hours to complete the project within the allotted timeframe.

The success of the conversion was a testament to the hard work and dedication of my team. We completed the project in just two months, a feat that was both impressive and rewarding. The new filing system streamlined operations and improved the overall efficiency of the medical records department.

Reflections on the Early Years

As I look back on my early years in Houston, I am struck by the contrast between the bustling city and the quiet moments of reflection and camaraderie. The experiences I had, from working with Cable Slabs to exploring the nightlife and enjoying weekends in Galveston, shaped my understanding of life and work.

Houston was a city of contrasts, a place where opportunity and challenge coexisted. The rapid growth and development of the city mirrored my own journey, as I navigated the demands of work, school, and personal life. The friendships I forged and the experiences I had during those early years were foundational to my growth and development.

The lessons learned in Houston, from the importance of hard work to the value of friendship and the joy of discovery, have stayed with me throughout my life. The city's energy and vibrancy were a reflection of my own aspirations and dreams, and the experiences I had during those formative years continue to inspire me to this day.

My friends and I would attend Astros games in the Astrodome whenever a good pitching matchup was scheduled. We would buy $3.00 cheap nosebleed seats and then moved down during the 3rd inning to better vacant seats.

One afternoon in Galveston, we were discussing how the Houston Oilers had just signed Earl Campbell. The following Monday, I stood in line for Season tickets. This worked out well as Rick, his Father, our friend Jim and myself would partake in Oiler home games.

I became an avid Astros and Oilers' fan.

Chapter VI
Devastation and Heartbreak

In the spring of 1977, my life was moving forward at a steady pace. I was working at Hermann Hospital in Houston, feeling secure in the path I was carving out for myself. I was building a life, thousands of miles away from my hometown of Poughkeepsie, with the intent of starting something new. Yet, in a way that life so often does, everything changed in an instant.

The Call

It was an ordinary morning at the hospital when I received a phone call from the Houston Police Department. The voice on the other end belonged to an HPD sergeant, calm but serious, telling me I needed to call my Uncle George back home in New York. His tone didn't reveal much, but I knew from the pit forming in my stomach that this was no routine call.

I hung up the phone and immediately dialed my uncle, my heart pounding as the seconds stretched out. When he answered, I could hear the struggle in his voice as he tried to find the words. "Fred," he said softly, "there's been an accident... Your mother and father perished in a house fire last night."

For a moment, the world seemed to stop. The noise of the hospital, the chaos of daily life—all of it faded into the background as those words echoed in my mind. My mother and father—gone, just like that.

I remember standing there, my knuckles white as I gripped the phone, disbelief clouding every thought. How could this be real? How could life, in one split second, change so dramatically?

Calling Friends

In the haze that followed the call, I knew I had to take action. I had to go home, face what had happened, and be there for my family. But I couldn't do it alone. I needed the support of my closest friends, Chuck and Jim. Without hesitation, I called them and shared the devastating news. They responded as only true friends do—without hesitation, they told me they were booking the next flight to New York.

I also called my cousin Nancy, who lived in New York with her husband John. They promised to pick me up at LaGuardia when I arrived, offering to take care of me in whatever way they could. Even in the midst of my grief, I was grateful for the people around me, those who, despite the miles between us, were willing to drop everything to be by my side.

The Quiet Flight

The flight back to New York felt like it lasted an eternity. I sat there, in a daze, surrounded by strangers who had no idea that my world had just been shattered. I didn't know how to process the flood of emotions swirling within me—anger, disbelief, confusion, and sorrow. The weight of the loss pressed heavily on me, yet I knew I had to hold myself together.

I was the eldest son. It was my responsibility to lead, to offer strength and guidance in the face of this tragedy. As much as I wanted to fall apart, I knew that my family would be looking to me for support, especially my younger brothers, Jack and Mike.

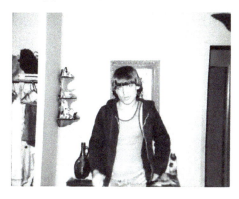
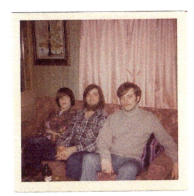

Mike *Mike, Jack, and Fred*

I kept replaying the phone call with my uncle in my mind, trying to make sense of the senseless. My parents, who had been a constant source of love and strength in my life, were gone, taken from me in the most sudden and cruel way imaginable.

Learning the Details

When I finally arrived in New York, Nancy and John were waiting for me at the airport. They embraced me with the kind of quiet understanding that words can't offer, then began filling me in on the events of that horrific night.

The fire had started in the early hours of May 15, 1977. My brother Mike, who was 16 at the time, had been home when it happened. He escaped by climbing out of his bedroom window and running to the neighbor's house. That neighbor, by some tragic twist of fate, was a firefighter. But by the time he returned to the house, it was too late.

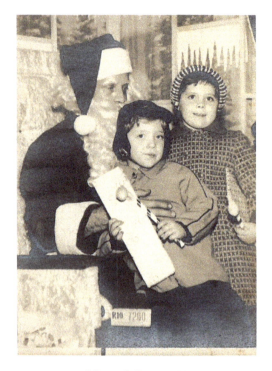

Me and Cousin Nancy

My parents had died of smoke inhalation. It was a bitter comfort to know that they hadn't suffered through the flames, but that knowledge did little to ease the sting of their loss. The fire had also taken my Aunt Janice, who had been visiting from Kingston. She'd suffered severe burns and passed away a few weeks later, another life claimed by the same tragedy.

The cause of the fire was never determined, though there were rumors it might have been the furnace. But in the end, it didn't matter. What mattered was that they were gone, and there was nothing I could do to bring them back.

A Premonition or Coincidence?

As we sat together, mourning the loss, I couldn't help but recall a dream I had just a few weeks before the fire. In that dream, I found myself standing over a coffin, looking at my father's face. He looked peaceful, serene. In the same dream appeared a friend I knew in High School named Stan. At the time, I thought nothing of it. Dreams are often just that—dreams. But the next day, I called home, concerned in a way that I couldn't explain.

My brother Jack had answered the phone, assuring me that everything was fine and that everyone was well. But just before we hung up, he mentioned something that made my heart skip a beat. "Oh, by the way," he said, almost as an afterthought, "I saw your old friend Stan the other day. He was asking about you."

I didn't think much of it then, but in light of what happened, I couldn't help but wonder if that dream had been a premonition of sorts. When I saw my father lying in the casket at the funeral home, he looked exactly as he had in my dream—calm, at peace. Whether it was mere coincidence or something more, I still don't know. But it has stayed with me all these years.

The Eulogy

For two weeks, I stayed with my Aunt Shirley and Uncle George in New York, trying to settle my parents' estate and wrap my mind around the enormity of their loss. The grief was overwhelming, but I knew that I had to be strong for my family, especially my brothers. Mike, who was still a minor, wanted to stay in Hyde Park and finish school with his friends. Jack had already moved out and was living on his own, but Mike needed someone to take care of him.

Uncle George and Aunt Shirley agreed to become Mike's guardians, and with that settled, we began the long and painful process of finalizing the estate. My parents hadn't left a will, so everything was to be divided equally between us three boys. I gave my share of the house to Jack and Mike. Jack rebuilt the house and eventually sold it, while Mike would have to wait until he was 18 to receive his inheritance.

During this time, I also wrote a eulogy for my parents—a final tribute to the two people who had given me life and love and shaped me into the person I had become.

Mom and Dad,

"You brought us into this world, you gave us love and understanding. You nurtured us and set us on the path to a wonderful life. With your guidance, you let us make our own choices. The right choices.

Mom and Dad, you have accomplished your earthly mission. Rest in peace."

Fred, Jack, and Mike

Writing those words was one of the hardest things I've ever done. How do you sum up a lifetime of love and sacrifice in just a few short sentences? But I hoped, in some small way, that they could hear me—that they knew how much they meant to me and how deeply they would be missed.

Finding Strength Amid Tragedy

As executor of the estate, I inherited my father's 1975 Dodge Dart Swinger. It wasn't much, but it was a piece of him that I could take with me back to Houston. I drove it all the way across the country, the miles stretching out before me as I tried to make sense of everything that had happened.

Throughout the ordeal, I felt like I was running on adrenaline, just as I had during the most intense moments of combat in Vietnam. It was as if my body went into survival mode, focusing on what needed to be done rather than the overwhelming grief threatening to consume me. In a strange way, my experiences with death and loss in the war had prepared me for this moment.

I was determined to honor my parents' memory by continuing to pursue my goals, finishing my degree, and building the life that they had always wanted for me. With the support of Uncle George, Aunt Shirley, Nancy, and John, I was able to survive this devastating chapter of my life. They were my rock, just as Jack and Mike were, and I loved them all deeply for standing by me during my darkest hours.

Moving Forward

The loss of my parents left a hole in my heart that could never truly be filled. There are days, even now, when I think of them and wish that I could pick up the phone, hear their voices, and tell them about the life I've built. I know they would be proud.

But in the end, I found a way to move forward. Not because the grief ever went away, but because I knew they would want me to live my life fully, to carry on the legacy of love and strength that they had passed down to me.

Their memory lives on in everything I do, and though their physical presence is gone, I carry them with me, always.

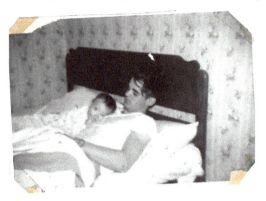

Me and Dad at home in Creek Road

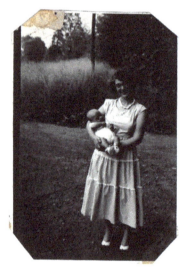

Me and Mom Creek Road

Chapter VII
Retail Credit at Joske's of Houston

1978-1981

The months following the tragedy of losing my parents were some of the hardest I had ever experienced. In the midst of the sorrow and the responsibility of settling the estate, I found myself at a crossroads. Life in Houston, though far from home, had begun to feel like a new start after the fire. Then, one phone call from my friend Rick would change everything, setting me on a course I hadn't anticipated.

A Job Offer and a Change of Direction

It was a humid evening in late 1978 when my phone rang. Rick, who had been one of my closest friends, was on the other end, his voice lively and full of excitement. "Fred, there's an opening at Joske's," he said. I had known Rick for years, and we had shared our fair share of beers and late-night conversations about life. He had been promoted to a supervisory role in New Accounts and now reported directly to the department manager. "I think you should come back to finance," Rick continued, his tone insistent. "This position could be a great fit for you."

At that moment, I hesitated. I had spent the past few years immersed in the world of medical records at Hermann Hospital. It had been rewarding, but after the emotional toll of my parents' passing, I wasn't sure if I was ready for a change—or if I had the energy to pursue one. But Rick was persuasive, as always. He convinced me to meet him for dinner at our favorite Mexican restaurant, promising to talk through everything.

Over enchiladas and margaritas, Rick made his case. "You've got a good head for finance," he told me. "This is a good opportunity, and it might be exactly what you need to get back on your feet." By the end of the meal, I had to admit that he was right. The routine and structure of the job were exactly what I needed to refocus my life. I agreed to take the job in New Accounts, knowing it was time to move forward and carve a new path for myself.

Settling Into the Role

The position at Joske's started as a part-time evening job. From 4 PM until the stores closed at 9, I worked in New Accounts, managing credit applications and helping customers navigate the process of opening lines of credit. It was a shift from my previous work, but I found the change refreshing. The structure of the job allowed me to take a break from school while still keeping myself busy during the evenings.

About six months into the job, Rick transitioned into a new role as the manager of the Authorizations Department, leaving his previous position in New Accounts open. With Rick's recommendation and the support of the New Accounts Manager, I was promoted to Rick's old job. We were once again working side by side, though now I had more responsibility. We spent our evenings managing the Credit Department, and our weekends enjoying trips to Rick's beach house. The camaraderie we had built over the years helped me stay grounded during a tumultuous time in my life.

But, as with many things in life, change was inevitable. Not long after settling into our roles at Joske's, Rick made the decision to leave the retail world behind for a career in the oil industry. His departure felt like the end of an era, but it also opened up new opportunities for me. Shortly after, I was recommended for Joske's Executive Training Program, a career-defining moment that fast-tracked my advancement within the company.

Rising Through the Ranks

I had always considered myself hardworking, but the Executive Training Program was a chance to prove myself in a new way. I was one of the first employees without a college degree to be accepted into the program, a fact that both humbled and motivated me. I knew that I would have to work twice as hard to earn the same respect as others, but I was determined to make the most of the opportunity.

After completing the program, I was promoted to Authorizations Manager, overseeing a team of eight employees. Our department was responsible for authorizing credit card transactions for all five Joske's locations in the area. If a credit card charge didn't go through, a call would flash on the register, and it was up to my team to evaluate the customer's credit and either approve or decline the purchase. The holiday season, in particular, was a whirlwind of activity. The pace was frenetic, but I thrived on the excitement. The ringing phones, the last-minute approvals, the constant flow of people—it all energized me in a way I hadn't expected.

However, not everything about the job was smooth sailing. One day, I discovered a fraudulent scheme involving one of my own employees. One of our authorization clerks had been approving charges on a friend's credit card, allowing them to make purchases they couldn't afford. It was a breach of trust, and as much as it pained me, I had no choice but to dismiss the clerk. It was a harsh reminder that, even in the most exciting roles, integrity was paramount.

Love and a New Beginning

Around the same time that I was promoted, another significant event occurred in my life—one that would shape the course of my personal life for years to come. One of the women who worked in my department handed in her resignation, and before she left, I mustered up the courage to ask her out on a date. We had always gotten along well at work, and there was something about her that made me want to know her better. Our first date was a success, and what started as a simple evening out soon blossomed into something deeper. We continued to see each other, and in 1980, we got married. Her name was Val, and she brought a sense of stability and warmth into my life that I hadn't realized I was missing.

Shortly after our wedding, Val became pregnant with our first child. I'll never forget her cravings for Big Macs—she couldn't seem to get enough of them. When our son, Sean, was born, it felt like a new chapter had begun. We were living in a cozy patio home in the suburbs of Houston, and Val's mother moved in with us to help with the baby. For a time, life felt settled, and the future seemed bright.

But Val had always dreamed of owning a horse, a dream she had carried with her since childhood. And as much as I loved our suburban life, I wanted to make her dream come true. So, we bought a beautiful Appaloosa horse named LaRainda—Rainy, for short. Rainy was a gentle creature, and Val adored her. We stabled her nearby, and for a while, it seemed like the perfect arrangement.

The Call of the Country Life

As much as we loved our little home in the suburbs, it didn't take long for us to realize that keeping Rainy stabled was becoming too expensive. Val and I began to dream of something more—something that would allow us to live a quieter life in the country while also providing the space we needed for our growing family.

After months of searching, we found the perfect place: a sprawling five-bedroom ranch house in Splendora, Texas. The property came with four acres of land, a barn, and plenty of room for all the animals we would eventually acquire. Before long, our ranch became home to not just Rainy, but also horses, a cow, a pig, turkeys, chickens, geese, and even a duck. It was a far cry from our suburban life, but it was everything we had dreamed of—and more.

Splendora was a quiet, unassuming town that bordered Cleveland, Texas. Life there moved at a slower pace, and we found ourselves adjusting to the rhythm of country living. One day, Val and I were out driving, looking for our local voting place, when we stumbled upon a trailer with a sign that simply said, "Vote here." It seemed like a quiet, unremarkable place—until we stepped out of the truck and were greeted by a man standing on a tree stump, shouting about the Democratic Party candidates.

As we stood there in bewilderment, the man began listing the candidates, one by one. But when he reached Jesse Jackson's name, his tone changed. "And if you vote for Jesse Jackson," he shouted, "we know where you live." Val and I exchanged glances and quickly got out of there, our nerves on edge. It was a strange, unsettling experience, but it was also a reminder of the complexities of small-town life.

Building a Future

As the years passed, our life in Splendora settled into a comfortable routine. We raised our animals, cared for our growing son, and worked to build a future that we could be proud of. My career at Joske's continued to progress, and though the demands of retail collections were tough, I found satisfaction in the challenge of my new role as assistant Collection Manager. We worked hard to collect past-due debts within 90 days, knowing that if we failed, the accounts would be handed off to outside collection agencies who would take a third of the money collected.

One of my responsibilities was to visit and monitor these outside agencies, ensuring that they were handling our accounts with care.

It wasn't an easy job, but it was one that I took seriously. Every day brought new challenges, but I faced them with the same determination that had carried me through the difficult times before.

As I look back on those years at Joske's, I can see how much they shaped me—both personally and professionally. It wasn't just about the work; it was about the relationships I built, the lessons I learned, and the life that Val and I created together. From the fast-paced world of retail credit to the quiet, peaceful days on our ranch in Splendora, every step of the journey was a reminder that life, in all its complexity, is about more than just the work we do. It's about the people we love, the dreams we pursue, and the choices we make along the way. And in those years, I learned that no matter where life takes us, it's the people and the dreams that matter most.

Chapter VIII
(Oil and Gas Credit)

A Call to Adventure

The phone call came on a warm afternoon in 1981, just as I was settling into my routine at Joske's. It was Rick, my old friend who had previously guided me through the maze of the retail world. I could sense the excitement in his voice, and it piqued my curiosity. "Fred," he said, "there's an opportunity in the oil and gas industry that I think you'd be perfect for. You should reach out to the Assistant Treasurer at Tomlinson Interests."

I had never considered a career in the oil patch, but the thought of a new challenge and a higher salary was enticing. With a growing family and bills to pay, the prospect of leaving retail for a position in a lucrative industry was hard to ignore.

I did as Rick suggested and called the Assistant Treasurer. The conversation flowed easily, and he asked me to come in for an interview. As I drove to Tomlinson's offices, a mix of excitement and nervousness washed over me. I was stepping into a world that was foreign yet tantalizing, where fortunes could be made and lost in the blink of an eye.

The Interview

Walking into the sleek, modern office of Tomlinson Interests felt surreal. The atmosphere was charged with ambition and energy, a stark contrast to the familiarity of Joske's. The office was adorned with artwork depicting oil rigs and vast fields of golden grass swaying under the Texas sun. I could hear the distant hum of conversations and the tapping of keyboards as professionals hustled through their day.

The interview went smoothly; I spoke confidently about my background in credit and collections and how my experience at Joske's had equipped me with the skills necessary for this new role. The Assistant Treasurer nodded appreciatively, his brow furrowing slightly as he considered my answers. "You seem like you understand the nuances of managing collections," he remarked. "This industry has its own challenges, but with your experience, I think you could fit in well."

When I left the building, I felt a thrill of hope. I was ready for a change, ready to dive into the challenges and rewards of the oil and gas industry. Just a few days later, I received the call that would alter my career path forever: I was offered the position of Credit and Collections Supervisor.

With my family's needs in mind, I jumped at the opportunity, ready to embrace this new chapter.

A Different Kind of Business

As I settled into my role at Tomlinson Interests, I quickly realized how different this industry was from retail. Deals were often done with a handshake, a nod of trust between parties. However, with the downturn in the market, companies were beginning to realize the stark reality of their outstanding receivables. The very foundations of the industry were shifting beneath us.

Tomlinson was primarily an Exploration and Production company, meaning we engaged with investors and Joint Owners who held working interests in exploratory wells. My job was to ensure that Joint Interest Billings, or JIBs, were collected promptly. For instance, if a Joint Owner had a 10% working interest in a well, (as set forth in the Joint Operating Agreement), they would be billed for 10% of the drilling and operating costs. When production began, they would receive 10% of the revenue generated from the well.

My role required working closely with various departments—Accounting, Land, and Legal—to navigate the complexities of the Joint Operating Agreements. These agreements designated the interest, payment timelines, and our rights as the Operator to offset revenues if necessary. It was a dance of sorts, requiring diplomacy, persistence, and a keen understanding of the nuances involved.

The communication skills I had honed in retail served me well here. I found it easier to collect from oil and gas companies who owned working interests than from individuals or trusts. There was a camaraderie in the industry, a shared understanding of the stakes involved.

The Highs of Success

The thrill of collecting millions of dollars in receivables was exhilarating. Each successful transaction felt like a victory, a testament to my hard work and determination. I was making a name for myself in the industry, becoming a go-to person for collections.

One day, I found myself in a particularly intense negotiation with a large company that had fallen behind on its payments. The stakes were high; this company held a significant interest in several wells, and their failure to pay would have a cascading effect on our cash flow. I prepared meticulously, reviewing every detail of our agreements, the costs incurred, and the revenue generated.

When I entered the conference room, the atmosphere was charged. Executives from both sides were present, and I could feel the tension in the air. After a few minutes of small talk, we dove into the details. I presented our case, outlining the obligations and the potential consequences of non-payment.

The discussions turned heated, but I maintained my composure, responding to objections with facts and figures. I could sense that the room was slowly shifting; the representatives from the other company began to acknowledge the validity of our claims. After what felt like hours, we reached an agreement that included a payment plan. As I walked out of that meeting, I felt elated. I had not only collected what was owed but had also established a valuable relationship with a key player in the industry.

I often worked late into the night, drafting emails and making phone calls to ensure payments were received on time. I thrived in this environment, relishing the challenges and the strategic thinking required. Each day presented new problems to solve, new negotiations to navigate.

But as much as I loved the adrenaline rush of my work, there were days when I felt the weight of the world on my shoulders. The stress of keeping the company's finances afloat during a downturn took its toll. I would come home exhausted, only to be met by the joyful chaos of my young family. Sean, now a toddler, brought light into our lives, and I cherished those moments. Val's warmth and understanding made the long hours bearable. She supported me in ways I couldn't always articulate, helping me to see the bigger picture even when the immediate stresses felt overwhelming.

The Unraveling

Yet, even in the midst of success, I began to notice signs that things were changing at Tomlinson. The company was making cuts, laying off key personnel, including the Treasurer and my boss, the Assistant Treasurer. The atmosphere that had once buzzed with energy began to feel strained, and whispers of impending layoffs circulated among my colleagues.

Despite my success in collecting debts, I couldn't shake the feeling that I was witnessing the beginning of the end for my role at the company. I tried to remain optimistic, telling myself that as long as I kept delivering results, my position would be secure. But deep down, I knew better.

During this period, I found myself retreating into my work, using it as a distraction from the uncertainty that loomed over us. Late nights became the norm, and I often found myself scrolling through reports long after my colleagues had gone home. I began to keep a close eye on our cash flow projections, worrying about the implications of each new delay in payments.

There were moments when I felt the walls closing in around me. One Friday evening, as I sat in my office, I received a call from a Joint Owner who was disputing a billing. The conversation quickly escalated into a heated exchange. I could feel my blood pressure rising as I struggled to keep my cool.

"Fred, I don't care what your invoices say," the owner snapped. "We don't owe you a dime until you prove that the well is producing!"

My heart raced as I listened to the accusations, but I remained calm. "I understand your frustration, and I'm more than willing to discuss this further," I replied, fighting to keep my voice steady. "But we have to adhere to the terms of the Joint Operating Agreement."

As I hung up the phone, I felt drained. The weight of the industry's volatility pressed heavily on my shoulders, and I wondered how long I could sustain this pace. It was a turning point, a moment when I began to realize that my emotional well-being was at stake.

Signs of Trouble

As the weeks progressed, the situation at Tomlinson grew more precarious. With the layoffs, the remaining staff were stretched thin, and the atmosphere of uncertainty began to affect morale. I watched as my colleagues exchanged nervous glances, their smiles fading as conversations turned to speculation about who would be next.

I started interviewing with Damson Oil Company, seeking to secure a safety net in case the inevitable happened. It was a difficult position to be in—trying to balance my current job while actively looking for a new one. I poured my heart and soul into my work, reminding myself that I had a family to support. I needed to stay focused, to keep pushing through the uncertainty.

Every time I entered the office, I felt a knot tighten in my stomach. The sense of camaraderie that had once filled the halls was replaced by an undercurrent of fear. One afternoon, I ran into Joan, a colleague I had worked closely with. Her eyes were red, and she looked exhausted.

"Hey, Fred," she said, her voice barely above a whisper. "Do you think we're safe? I keep hearing rumors."

I wanted to reassure her, to say that everything would be okay, but I couldn't bring myself to lie. "I don't know, Joan. But let's keep working hard and hope for the best."

The uncertainty gnawed at me, and I found myself questioning every decision I had made to pursue this career. Was the risk worth it? Would I be able to provide for my family if the worst happened?

The Layoff

It was a fateful Friday afternoon when I Returned from a collection run to one of our gas pipeline purchasers. With a $5 Million check in hand, I presented it to our CFO who said "nice collection work"!

"Fred, I'm sorry to inform you that due to ongoing financial constraints, we have to let you go."

My heart sank. I sat in stunned silence, the weight of the news crashing over me. I had poured everything into this job, and now it was gone. I felt a mix of anger, sadness, and fear—a cacophony of emotions swirling within me.

I took a moment to collect myself. The office that had once felt like a second home now felt cold and unwelcoming. I gathered my belongings, the memories of my time at Tomlinson flashing through my mind. The friendships I had forged, the victories I had celebrated, the challenges I had overcome—all of it felt like a dream now.

When I walked out of the building, I felt as though I was leaving a piece of myself behind. I had invested so much time and energy into this role, and now I was stepping into an uncertain future.

The Fallout

As I drove home, I replayed the events of the past months in my mind. The layoffs, the whispers of trouble, the tension in the air—it all made sense now, but it didn't soften the blow. I arrived home and found Val in the kitchen, her face lighting up at the sight of me.

"Fred! You're home early!"

Her excitement was palpable, but the weight of my news hung heavily in the air. I took a deep breath, steeling myself for the moment. "Val, we need to talk."

Her smile faded as she sensed the seriousness in my tone. "What's wrong?"

I sat down at the kitchen table and shared the news, watching as her expression shifted from concern to shock. "Oh, Fred, I'm so sorry!" she exclaimed, her voice filled with empathy. "What are we going to do?"

The reality of the situation hit us both like a ton of bricks. We had bills to pay, a mortgage to cover, and a young son who relied on us. I felt a knot forming in my stomach as the enormity of our situation began to sink in.

Val wrapped her arms around me, and I allowed myself to lean into her embrace. In that moment, I realized how much I needed her support. She was my anchor, and together we would find a way through this storm.

Navigating the Unknown

The next few weeks were a blur of uncertainty. I spent hours updating my resume and networking with contacts I had made over the years. I applied for positions that piqued my interest, but each rejection stung more than the last. The fear of not being able to provide for my family loomed large in my mind.

Despite the pressure, I was determined to keep my spirits up. I channeled my energy into job searching, but I also made sure to be present for Val and Sean. I wanted to show them that, even in difficult times, we could find joy in the little things.

We began to explore local parks, take family walks, and even indulge in ice cream outings. Sean's laughter became a balm for my soul, reminding me of what truly mattered. Each day, I found comfort in the mundane: cooking dinner, helping Sean with his toys, and sharing stories with Val.

I also kept in touch with my old colleagues, exchanging updates and insights about job openings. While still at Tomlinson, one day, I received a call from Rick, who had been keeping tabs on my situation. "Fred, I have a lead for you. Damson is looking for someone in their credit department. I think you'd be a great fit!"

His encouragement reignited a spark within me. I applied immediately and landed an interview, a glimmer of hope shining through the haze of uncertainty.

New Beginnings

The interview at Damson Oil Company was different from my previous experiences. The atmosphere was relaxed, and the executives seemed genuinely interested in getting to know me. I spoke candidly about my journey, my successes, and the lessons I had learned along the way.

As the interview progressed, I felt a renewed sense of purpose. This was my chance to leverage my experience and step back into the industry with a fresh perspective.

Weeks passed, and just as I was beginning to lose hope, I received the call I had been waiting for: I was offered the position at Damson. The relief washed over me like a wave, and I immediately shared the news with Val.

We celebrated that night with a simple dinner at home, a reminder that we could find joy even in the face of adversity. I felt a sense of gratitude wash over me—gratitude for my family, for the opportunity to start anew, and for the resilience I had developed through this journey.

Embracing the Future

As I began my new role at Damson, I carried with me the lessons learned from my time at Tomlinson. The challenges I faced had shaped me, but they hadn't broken me. I approached my work with a renewed sense of determination, eager to make a difference in my new position.

I was ready to embrace the opportunities ahead, knowing that, regardless of what lay in store, I had the strength to navigate whatever challenges came my way. The experience had been a crucible, forging resilience and instilling a deeper appreciation for the bonds of family and the importance of perseverance.

As I reflected on my journey, I knew that my story was far from over. It was merely the next chapter, a new beginning filled with promise and hope.

Chapter IX
Damson Oil Corporation (1982-1985)

A New Beginning

In 1982, I found myself stepping into a new role at Damson Oil Corporation as the Credit and Collection Supervisor. It felt like a fresh start after the upheavals I had experienced in my earlier career. This was not just another job; it was an opportunity to create a credit function from the ground up—a one-man shop for the collection of Joint Interest and Revenue Receivables. The responsibility felt heavy, but it also ignited a fire within me. I had a chance to make a significant impact, and I was determined to seize it.

Damson Oil was headquartered in New York City, a hub of real estate and oil and gas operations. Ironically, the Treasurer at headquarters had been a roommate of Roger Staubach during their days at the Naval Academy. While I didn't share that illustrious connection, I was ready to carve out my own legacy within the company.

I quickly got to work screening potential creditworthy Joint Partners. I remember my first day vividly—papers scattered across my new desk, the hum of the office around me, and the thrill of the unknown. It was both exhilarating and terrifying. But as the days turned into weeks, I began to find my rhythm, and I was soon able to report back to the Controller with good news—collecting millions of dollars and significantly reducing Damson's receivable exposure.

Each success fueled my determination, a testament to my commitment to the company.

Family Milestones

In the midst of my professional accomplishments, life at home was equally transformative. In the summer of 1982, Val and I welcomed our daughter, Heather, into the world. The joy of becoming a father for the second time filled our home with a warmth that overshadowed the challenges we faced. I could often hear Val softly singing to Heather during those late-night feedings, her voice soothing and filled with love. I cherished those moments, standing at the doorway and watching them bond.

As I juggled my responsibilities at Damson, I was also filled with pride every time I received praise from the Controller. He often asked me what I had collected that day, eager for good news to relay back to headquarters. I wore those moments like armor against the stress of the job, knowing that my hard work was recognized and valued. I felt like I was contributing not just to my family but also to something larger, something that mattered.

The Storm

However, life is never without its storms—both literal and metaphorical. In 1984, Hurricane Alicia struck, wreaking havoc across Houston. The winds howled like a banshee, and I could hear the crack of trees falling outside from Alicia's spin off tornados . I remember standing with Sean, peering through the living room picture window, our eyes wide with fear as we watched nature unleash its fury.

Suddenly, a tree loomed above us, seemingly headed straight for our home. In a split second, I snatched Sean into my arms and sprinted toward the back of the house, where Val and Heather were huddled together. The wind howled around us as we stayed close, praying for safety during the onslaught.

The damage was catastrophic. We lost over 30 / 60-foot oak trees, some of which crashed onto our property. One tree fell on the corner of our living room, and another obliterated Val's car. The sight of those grand oaks lying like toothpicks sent a chill down my spine, a haunting reminder of how quickly things could change.

In the aftermath, we were left without electricity for two long weeks. The barn sustained extensive damage, and the repairs seemed overwhelming. Thankfully, my brother Jack lived in Houston and, along with his friend, was able to help us rebuild. Jack's brother-in-law Otis brought along ice from his work at Texas DOT, a simple but essential lifeline during those sweltering days without power. The chaos of the storm contrasted sharply with the tenderness of family life, leaving me torn between gratitude for our safety and despair over the destruction surrounding us.

A Shift in Seasons

As the months passed, I continued to thrive at Damson, my successes paving the way for new opportunities. I would later apply my expertise at three more Independent Exploration and Production

Companies, starting with Monsanto Oil Company, a subsidiary of Monsanto Chemical. However, this time, the stakes felt even higher.

Monsanto Oil was in the midst of being acquired by BHP Petroleum, an Australian oil company, and I was brought on as a contractor with no guarantees for the future. The stress of that uncertainty weighed heavily on my shoulders. Every day felt like walking a tightrope, a precarious balance between hope and fear. I often found solace in the knowledge that I had made a name for myself at Damson, but the looming acquisition kept me on edge.

Then came the moment of reprieve. Thankfully, BHP hired me, and I spent the next eight years in a position that allowed me to flourish. I remember teaching our Australian CEO how to play horseshoes during company picnics. It was a small moment of levity amid the pressures of corporate life, a reminder that laughter can bridge even the widest cultural divides.

The Fraying Threads

While my professional life was stabilizing, my personal life was unraveling. In 1987, Val and I decided to divorce after years of drifting apart. It was a decision rooted in the changes we had both undergone—particularly after our children, Sean and Heather, began grade school. The pressures of commuting 60+ miles for work each day had strained our relationship, with me working at BHP in Southwest Houston and Val commuting to Anadarko Petroleum in North Houston as a Geology Tech.

I watched as Val thrived in her new role, making friends quickly, and I felt a pang of sadness mixed with pride. Our life together had changed so drastically, and as we both navigated our new paths, the weight of our commitments to work and family pressed on us. Our once-close relationship seemed overshadowed by the distance created by our careers.

Even though we were living in the same town, our lives had taken different trajectories, and it was becoming increasingly difficult to maintain our connection. I felt the void of her absence deeply, a stark contrast to the warmth we had shared in our early years. I often found myself reminiscing about our happier times, longing for the intimacy we had lost.

The Journey Back to School

After my time at BHP, I sought new opportunities and interviewed with Apache Corporation. Unfortunately, they required a college degree, a barrier I had not anticipated. Faced with the reality of needing further education, I took a leap of faith. I enrolled in a government program designed to assist displaced workers in re-education and entering new careers.

Returning to school was both exhilarating and daunting. I was filled with a mix of excitement and anxiety as I walked through the halls of the institution. I was surrounded by younger students who seemed so sure of their paths, and I couldn't help but wonder if I was out of my depth. However, I clung to the belief that education could open new doors, providing me with the skills I needed to advance my career.

The classroom became a space of rediscovery for me. I immersed myself in my studies, fueled by a determination to provide for my children and myself. I learned to embrace the discomfort of the unknown, pushing through self-doubt to forge a new identity—one that was resilient and adaptable. Each late night spent studying and every paper I wrote became a building block, reinforcing my commitment to my family's future.

New Opportunities

My time at school was not without its challenges, but I was resolute. The knowledge I gained became a beacon of hope, guiding me toward new career paths. I re-entered the job market with renewed vigor, armed with new skills and a determination to succeed.

As I reflect on those years at BHP and beyond, I realize that every experience—both good and bad—shaped who I was becoming. The trials of the hurricane, the joy of family milestones, the pressures of work, and the pains of divorce all contributed to my growth. I emerged from that period not just as a survivor but as someone who had learned to navigate the complexities of life with resilience.

Moving Forward

While my relationship with Val had changed, the love for our children remained a strong foundation. As we transitioned into our new roles as co-parents, I recognized that our shared commitment to Sean and Heather would always bind us together. In the end, it was about ensuring their happiness and well-being, a priority that transcended our differences.

The journey through those years was a crucible, testing my strength and resolve. Yet, as I stepped into new roles and responsibilities, I felt a renewed sense of purpose and hope. The challenges I faced—whether at Damson or later at Monsanto and BHP—only served to reinforce my belief in the power of perseverance.

As I closed this chapter of my life, I looked forward with optimism, ready to embrace whatever lay ahead. The lessons I learned would carry me through the uncertain waters of the future, and I was confident that, with each new opportunity, I would continue to grow, adapt, and thrive.

Chapter X
My Blended Family

In 1990, after the tumultuous years of my first marriage, I found a fresh start in the most unexpected of places. I had recently gone through a painful divorce and was seeking solace in travel, planning a solo trip to clear my mind. I walked into a travel agency in Houston with the intention of booking my escape, but instead, I met someone who would forever change the course of my life. Her name was Lene, a bright and confident Filipina woman who had a spark of life in her eyes that drew me in instantly.

Lene had her own story to tell. Originally from the Philippines, she had once owned her own travel agency back in Manila before making her way to the U.S. We hit it off right from the start, the ease of our conversation was undeniable, and before I knew it, I was asking her to dinner. That one meal turned into several, and soon, the trip I had planned to take alone became unnecessary—I had already embarked on the most important journey of my life, one that involved her.

With the severance pay I had received from BHP, I helped Lene start a travel agency here in Houston, specializing in flights to and from Manila. Her main clients were Filipinos living in the U.S., yearning to reconnect with their homeland. Lene was sharp, organized, and passionate about her business, and I did what I could to support her, often delivering tickets while I was finishing my degree. As a bonus, with all the complimentary flights and hotel stays we earned through the business, we traveled extensively—both domestically and internationally. From the sun-kissed beaches of the Caribbean to the bustling streets of New York City, we shared countless adventures, creating memories I would cherish for a lifetime.

Welcoming a New Family

Marrying Lene didn't just bring me a new partner in life; it also gave me the gift of a new family. She had three teenagers from her previous marriage: Marc, Anna, and Maria. From the moment I met them, I knew I wanted to be more than just their stepfather—I wanted to be a father to them in every sense of the word. Sean and Heather, my children from my first marriage, began spending weekends with us, and just like that, we were one big, blended family.

For the most part, the kids were well-adjusted to our new life together. The girls, Anna and Maria, became fast friends with Sean and Heather, while Marc found a place in the brotherhood of sorts that he formed with Sean. I gave the boys free reign of the garage, which soon became their own little haven. They turned it into the neighborhood bicycle repair shop and worked on whatever bizarre projects they could dream up. One day it was a broken lawnmower, the next, they were constructing a go-kart from spare parts they found in the garage and in the local junkyards. The garage became their kingdom, and I encouraged their creativity as long as they stayed within certain boundaries.

Our neighborhood, in the southwest part of Houston, was diverse, with families from all over the world. Down the street lived a group of older boys whose father happened to be the Iraqi Consul General. Despite the differences in culture, the kids bonded over shared mischief. Every New Year's Eve and Fourth of July, they would compete with the Iraqi boys to see who could create the loudest fireworks display. It was a sight to behold, watching them stand shoulder to shoulder as they gleefully debated the merits of their latest concoction.

"Dad, I swear, this one's going to be the loudest yet!" Sean would declare, eyes alight with excitement.

Marc, nodding in agreement, would add, "The Iraqis won't know what hit them."

Of course, as a parent, I couldn't allow them to play with fire—literally—unsupervised. I set strict parameters and made sure to monitor their every move. They were only allowed one shot to execute their 'masterpiece,' and while I could see the thrill in their eyes, I also made sure they understood the importance of safety. But these were the moments that made me feel like we were building something solid as a family. The laughter, the small victories, the shared moments of joy—it was all starting to feel real and deeply rewarding.

Trouble at the Homestead

But life, as I had come to learn, is rarely without its share of heartache and trials. One day while I was working at BHP, I received a phone call that no parent ever wants to get. Lene's mother, who lived nearby, called me in a state of panic. Maria had called her, hysterical, saying that Anna's boyfriend had broken into our house through the garage and abducted her at gunpoint. My heart dropped.

I immediately called the County Sheriff's Office and reported the break-in and abduction. After that, I drove home faster than I ever had before, my mind racing with every terrifying possibility. The house was eerily quiet when I arrived, and all I could do was wait for law enforcement to arrive.

It seemed like hours before the Sheriff's deputy pulled into the driveway, though in reality, it had probably only been minutes. He took my statement, but I could see from his expression that he was not moving with the urgency I felt the situation deserved. While we were still talking, Lene and her sister, Vicky, arrived. The atmosphere was tense, with worry etched on all of our faces.

Then, as if by a miracle, a car pulled up out front. Anna emerged, her face streaked with tears, running toward us. She was safe—at least physically. She was sobbing uncontrollably as we rushed to get her inside. My relief was immediate, but it was soon overshadowed by anger. I turned to the deputy, incredulous.

"Aren't you going to go after him?" I demanded.

The deputy shook his head. "No, sir, we'll wait. We need to do this by the book."

My blood boiled at the calmness of his response, but I knew better than to push it further at that moment. All that mattered was getting Anna to safety and making sure she received the care she needed.

A Family Shattered

At the hospital, they processed a rape kit and kept Anna's clothing for forensic evidence. It was a gut-wrenching ordeal, watching this vibrant, beautiful girl I had come to love be subjected to such an invasion. Lene was beside herself, tears flowing freely, while Maria stood by, silent but clearly shaken. I did my best to hold everyone together, even though inside, I felt like I was falling apart. The whole night felt surreal, like a nightmare I couldn't wake up from.

Later that evening, after Anna had been checked out and had given her statement to the police, I sat her down and tried to talk to her about what had happened. She was hesitant to press charges, overwhelmed by the trauma and the fear.

"I can't… I can't do it. He said he'd kill you and Mom if I talked," she whispered, eyes downcast, trembling.

I took her hand, squeezing it tightly. "Anna, listen to me," I said, my voice firm but gentle. "No one terrorizes this family. We have to press charges. We have to stand up to him. You're not alone in this—I promise you that."

The next day, a Harris County detective came to our house to take Anna's statement. We told him that Ed, her boyfriend, was a Philippine national, that we knew where he worked, and even where his family lived. Anna bravely recounted the threats he had made, including the chilling promise that if she ever told anyone what had happened, he would kill both Lene and me.

The detective, a grizzled veteran of the force, looked Anna in the eye before leaving and said, "He might get away with this in the Philippines, but he's not getting away with it here."

It was a small comfort, but it meant the world to us in that moment.

A Threat Neutralized

Anna had met Ed at her 16th birthday party. At 22, he was older, more experienced, and had a way of manipulating her that we hadn't recognized at first. By the time she realized he wasn't the right person for her, it was already too late. She wanted to break up with him, but he refused to accept it. His possessiveness grew until it culminated in that horrific night.

After the threats to our family, I called my brother Jack and his wife, Donna. Without hesitation, they agreed to take the kids for a few days until the police could capture Ed. I'll never forget the wave of relief that washed over me when I got the call three days later, letting me know that Ed had been arrested at his place of employment. I could finally breathe again, knowing that he was behind bars.

However, the nightmare wasn't over. Just days after his arrest, Ed's family—led by his sister—came to Lene's travel agency, pleading with us to drop the charges. Their words were desperate, their pleas tugging at our hearts, but my resolve never wavered.

"If this had happened to your daughter," I told them, my voice steady and unwavering, "what would you do?"

They had no answer for that. They left the agency in silence, and we never heard from them again.

Anna's Bravery

The court case was grueling, but Anna's courage was nothing short of inspiring. She testified against Ed, despite the fear that he had instilled in her. Seeing her take the stand, watching her confront the man who had caused her so much pain, filled me with immense pride. It was one of the hardest things I had ever witnessed, but it was also one of the most powerful.

In the end, justice prevailed. Ed was sentenced to eight years in a Texas penitentiary. It wasn't enough, in my opinion, but it was something. More importantly, it marked the beginning of Anna's healing process. She had survived, and she had taken back control of her life.

Life after the trial wasn't easy. There were moments when the weight of what had happened seemed almost unbearable, but as a family, we leaned on each other. The bond between Lene and me grew even stronger, as did my relationship with each of the kids.

In the years that followed, we continued to navigate the challenges of our blended family. There were highs and lows, moments of joy and sorrow, but through it all, we remained united. The love that bound us together was stronger than anything life could throw at us, and in that love, we found the strength to heal.

I'll always remember those years as some of the most difficult but also the most meaningful. They taught me what it truly means to be a father, a husband, and a protector. They showed me that family isn't just about blood—it's about the people who stand by you, who lift you up when you're down, and who love you, unconditionally, through it all.

Thank you, Dad

"You became our guide and our light

Alongside our mother

You helped us to right

What we thought of or expect in a father

You changed our distrust

That we'll never feel the love of a father

You filled the void that we felt

When we were much younger

For the rest of our lives,

You'll forever be our father

For in this whole world,

We will choose no other.

Thank you for the privilege

Of letting us call you Dad.

We say it with Pride and Love

Coz you're our Angel sent

From Heaven above.

I love you Dad!

-Anna

My Endless Pride

Sean attended the University of Houston until he was hired as a warehouse supervisor for a nut and candy company in Houston. Sean's wife Dazzia is an independent Insurance Agent. Heather graduated from Texas A & M with a teaching degree. She taught 3rd graders for a couple of years. The kids were unruly, and the parents didn't give a darn. Her and her husband Nathan, now have a lucrative vending machine business and service almost all of the Texas' correctional facilities.

Marc did not attend college, but he prospered in Graphic Arts and Design. Anna graduated from my alma matter, The University of Houston – Downtown. She worked in Accounting for Houston's ABC affiliate and now works at the local FOX affiliate. Maria graduated from Texas Women's College and works in Finance.

I am so proud of all my kids. We must have done something right.

Unfortunately, after 25 years of marriage, Lene and I divorced in 2016.

Chapter XI
Apache Corporation (1997 -2019)

After graduation I was hired by the accounting firm of Horn-Wallce-Cole LLC. I worked for Randall Wallace and was assigned to Apache Corporation. I collected revenue receivables and whatever projects were assigned. Unfortunately, Randy contracted cancer and passed away rather suddenly. Apache had a position open as JIB Collection Supervisor. I was asked to apply by the Assistant Controller. I applied and was accepted. I started the collection process with 3 employees, and we worked in high dollar accounts first, then down to the low dollar accounts. I had them make folders on each account they worked on and document their conversations with Joint Interest Owners.

This was a tried-and-true method I employed everywhere I worked. I recommended that we form a Credit Committee that would meet once a month with our Land, Legal, and Accounting Departments to resolve any issues that came up after reviewing our high dollar accounts.

In 2000, I was asked to work in our Canada office in Calgary. I used my tried-and-true method with the assistance of 2 temporary employees. I arrived at the end of October, and we met our goal by the end of November. I stayed in Calgary through April 2001 until we hired a person to take my place.

Lake Louise

I would take weekend trips to Lake Louise and hike the trail that goes around the Lake and ends at the Glacier. On one such journey, I was alone and there were very few people at the Lake. There was fresh fallen snow with only my footprints going up the trail. I reached the half way point and decided to turn around and go back when I saw two sets of tracks in the snow. My tracks were clearly visible as well as Mountain Lion tracks that followed me up the trail. Probably thought I was too big to haul back to it's den.

After Calgary, Lene and I took a trip to Egypt. We did the Nile Cruise stopping at Luxor along the way to the Aswan Dam. We visited the Pyramids and the Cairo Museum as well. Our trip was before the Arab Spring. On the way home, we stopped in Hong Kong and did some shopping. We stayed with Lene's family in Manila and flew home from there.

When we started marketing our own gas, I helped start the Gas Marketing credit function. I developed a screening and financial analysis process of reviewing potential buyers and was successful in developing a portfolio of credit worthy purchasers. I worked closely with the Marketing and Legal Departments and negotiated the credit sections of gas purchase agreements and contracts with purchasers.

Chapter XII
Enron

The Early Whispers

The year 2001 was marked by economic turbulence that many businesses, large and small, could feel rumbling beneath their feet. But in the bustling halls of Apache Corporation, the oil and gas giant where I worked, the atmosphere remained characteristically focused and industrious. I had carved out a career for myself in the industry, drawing upon years of experience and a resilient spirit forged through personal trials and professional challenges. This particular chapter of my life, however, was set to test my mettle in ways I had never anticipated.

It was early October when the first whispers of trouble began to circulate about Enron Corporation, a company we had been dealing with regularly. The media started to trickle out stories suggesting financial irregularities, and there was a growing sense of unease. Enron, once a paragon of innovation and profitability in the energy sector, was suddenly under a dark cloud of suspicion. As the reports became more frequent, I could sense that something was gravely amiss.

Raising the Red Flag

As the Senior Treasury Advisor responsible for the Credit side of our sales agreements, I paid close attention to these developments. Our dealings with Enron were not insignificant as relayed to me by Apache's Oil Marketing Manager; we sold oil to them on a monthly basis. My gut instinct told me to dig deeper, so I started scrutinizing our transactions and the market reports with a keener eye. It became increasingly clear that Enron was teetering on the edge of a precipice.

I decided it was time to raise a red flag. I composed a memo detailing my concerns, emphasizing the growing risk of continuing our oil deliveries to Enron given their unstable situation. The potential fallout from their financial collapse could be catastrophic, not just for Enron but for any company entangled in their dealings. With a sense of urgency, I sent the memo up the chain of command, hoping it would reach someone who understood the gravity of the situation.

The memo did not stop at the mid-management level as I initially expected. Instead, it climbed higher and higher, eventually landing on the desk of Raymond Plank, Apache's CEO and Chairman of the Board. Plank was known for his sharp business acumen and no-nonsense approach, and I knew that if anyone could understand the implications, it would be him.

The Threat from Enron

Days passed in a tense blur. I focused on my work, but my mind was constantly churning with thoughts about the possible repercussions. Then, one morning, my phone rang. The voice on the other end was steely and unmistakably angry.

"This is , Chief Legal Counsel for Enron. I've just been informed of your proposal to halt deliveries. This is unacceptable and a breach of our sales agreements. We will pursue legal action if necessary."

The threat was real, and the tone made it clear that they were prepared to fight. I felt a chill run down my spine but also a surge of determination. The evidence was on our side, and I believed in the integrity of my decision.

"Mr. Derrick," I responded calmly, "We are acting in the best interest of Apache Corporation. Given the current uncertainties surrounding Enron, it would be irresponsible for us to continue without reevaluating the situation."

The call ended with no resolution, leaving a heavy sense of foreboding. For the next few days, the tension was palpable as we waited for the other shoe to drop. I kept my team informed, urging them to stay vigilant and prepare for any fallout. It was during these moments of uncertainty that the true strength of a team is revealed, and I was proud of how they rallied together.

The Collapse of Enron

Then, in December 2001, the news broke: Enron had filed for bankruptcy. The once-mighty corporation had crumbled under the weight of its own deceit and mismanagement. The scandal rocked the financial world, leaving a trail of devastation in its wake. But amidst the chaos, one thing was clear: we had made the right call. By halting our oil deliveries, we had shielded Apache from potentially disastrous financial losses. The company saved approximately $hundreds of thousands USD, a figure that spoke volumes about the importance of timely and informed decision-making.

Reflections on the Crisis

The aftermath of Enron's collapse was a sobering period. There was no sense of triumph, only a quiet acknowledgment of having navigated a perilous situation with caution and foresight. For me, it was a moment of reflection. The oil and gas industry, much like life itself, is fraught with risks and uncertainties. Success often hinges on the ability to make tough decisions and to stand by them, even in the face of adversity.

In the months that followed, Apache continued to thrive, and our actions during the Enron debacle were seen as a testament to our resilience and strategic thinking. It was a hard-earned lesson in the value of vigilance and the courage to act on one's convictions. As I moved forward in my career, this experience remained a touchstone, a reminder of the importance of integrity and the strength that comes from standing firm in the face of challenges.

Personal Impact and Professional Growth

The Enron episode was not just a corporate saga; it was a deeply personal journey. It tested my resolve and reaffirmed my belief in doing what is right, no matter the opposition. This experience shaped my professional ethos, teaching me that true leadership often involves making unpopular decisions and facing the consequences with dignity.

On a personal level, the crisis at Enron reminded me of the fragile nature of human endeavors. It was a stark illustration of how quickly fortunes can change and how crucial it is to remain grounded and principled. The lessons I learned during this period were invaluable, not only for my career but for my personal growth as well.

Building a Legacy

Looking back now, the Enron chapter is one of the many that shaped my journey, reinforcing the values that have guided me through the ups and downs of both personal and professional life. It is a story of caution, courage, and the unyielding spirit that drives us to navigate even the most treacherous waters with a steady hand and a clear vision.

My experiences with Enron also reinforced my commitment to fostering a culture of transparency and accountability within my team. I made it a point to share the lessons learned with my colleagues, encouraging open dialogue and proactive risk management. This approach not only strengthened our team but also contributed to a more resilient and adaptive organizational culture at Apache.

The Road Ahead

As I continued my career at Apache, the Enron debacle remained a pivotal moment in my professional narrative. It served as a constant reminder of the importance of ethical decision-making and the long-term benefits of maintaining integrity in the face of short-term pressures. These principles guided me through subsequent challenges and opportunities, shaping my contributions to the industry and my legacy as a leader.

In the end, the story of Enron is not just a tale of corporate failure and scandal. It is also a testament to the resilience of those who navigate the fallout with integrity and resolve. For me, it was a defining chapter that reinforced the core values that have driven my personal and professional journey.

As I reflect on this chapter of my life, I am grateful for the lessons learned and the strength gained from facing such formidable challenges. The Enron crisis was a crucible that tested my character and ultimately shaped me into a more thoughtful, principled, and resilient individual. And for that, I will always be thankful.

Lessons for Future Generations

The Enron scandal and its aftermath serve as a cautionary tale for future generations of business leaders and professionals. It underscores the importance of vigilance, ethical decision-making, and the courage to act in the face of uncertainty. By sharing my experiences, I hope to inspire others to uphold these values and navigate their own challenges with integrity and determination.

In sharing this story, I also aim to highlight the significance of teamwork and collective resilience. The support and dedication of my colleagues at Apache were instrumental in weathering the storm, and their contributions should not be overlooked. Together, we demonstrated that even in the darkest of times, a united and principled team can emerge stronger and more determined than ever.

A Final Reflection

As I bring this chapter to a close, I am reminded of the words of Winston Churchill: "Success is not final, failure is not fatal: It is the courage to continue that counts." The Enron saga was a profound lesson in the importance of perseverance and the enduring strength of the human spirit. It is a chapter that I will carry with me always, a testament to the power of integrity and the resilience that defines us all.

Although Enron was one of many in our portfolio of Oil and Gas Purchasers there are times when there are large transactions that must be scrutinized and where the understanding of our counterparts is key. Looking at payment histories and personal contact conversations can identify a purchaser who has been creditworthy but is having difficulty in the current economy. Satisfactory arrangements can be explored to prevent a bankruptcy filing. You do not need to force someone into bankruptcy if it can be avoided.

And so, as I look back on the journey that brought me through the tumultuous times of Enron and beyond, I am filled with a deep sense of gratitude and resolve. For it is through these trials that we discover our true strength and forge the path to a future defined by courage, integrity, and unwavering determination.

While at Apache, I was tasked with reviewing our Accounts Payable Vendors for authenticity and fraud prevention. I uncovered a Fraud that originated out of one of our field offices in Louisiana.

After reviewing invoices and research, I found that the Vendor was listed as a private farm operation. The invoice was for well services at one of our drilling locations. This raised major red flags in my mind. I immediately contacted the Field Office Manager who signed off on the invoice who said he will take a look at it and get back with me. He mentioned that the vendor was a reputable person in the local community. I then issued a memo to my chain of command including our Legal and Accounting departments.

It was discovered that the employee who submitted the work order invoices listed his neighbor's farm as the Vendor performing the work. We discovered invoices for thousands of dollars over a period of several months. It was further discovered that the Field Manager had signed a stack of work orders. It did not take much ingenuity or brain power on the part of the perpetrator to understand that all he had to do was fill in the blanks of the pre-approved work order invoice

The employee was also found to be driving with a suspended drivers license in an Apache vehicle. He would share the proceeds of their fraud scheme with his neighbor listed as a vendor.

It was a satisfying feeling uncovering this fraud and saving Apache thousands of dollars in possible future loses. As a result, Apache completely revamped their Vendor approval process.

Chapter XIII
Hurricane Katrina (2005)

The Calm Before the Storm

It was the end of August 2005, and while the summer heat in Texas felt unrelenting, there was an unusual stillness in the air. Little did I know, the true storm was brewing hundreds of miles away in the Gulf of Mexico. As I flipped through channels one evening, the news anchor's voice caught my attention. A hurricane, stronger than anything I had seen in years, was rapidly intensifying and barreling toward New Orleans.

The name Katrina was mentioned over and over, accompanied by images of darkening skies, towering waves, and hurried evacuations. The warnings became more urgent. They spoke of a monster storm, a hurricane so large and powerful that it was expected to bring untold devastation to the Gulf Coast. It wasn't long before the reports started showing images of people cramming into the Superdome—New Orleans' supposed refuge from the coming storm.

Katrina made landfall on August 29, 2005, and the devastation it left in its wake was unimaginable. The levees failed, the city flooded, and chaos ensued. For days, the news showed images of entire neighborhoods submerged under murky, contaminated waters. Families huddled on rooftops, waving for help, surrounded by debris and the remnants of their homes. It was one of the most heart-wrenching scenes I had ever witnessed.

The once lively streets of New Orleans were drowned, and in the hours after the storm, the true scale of the disaster unfolded. The Superdome, thought to be a place of refuge, became overwhelmed with evacuees. Tens of thousands of people—men, women, children, the elderly, the sick—packed into the massive stadium, but the conditions were deplorable. The news spoke of unbearable heat, lack of sanitation, insufficient food and water. And this was just the beginning.

As I watched the aftermath unfold from the safety of my Houston home, my heart ached for the people of New Orleans. Memories of my time as a medic in Vietnam flooded back—memories of chaos, of people in desperate need, and of my role in doing what I could to help. It had been years since I was last called upon to offer my medical experience, but in that moment, I knew what I had to do.

A Call to Action

The American Red Cross put out an urgent call for volunteers—especially those with medical experience. Houston, with its proximity and resources, was mobilizing quickly to help the flood victims. The Astrodome, which had long been retired as a sports venue, was now being offered as a refuge for those displaced by Katrina.

Without hesitation, I decided to help. Lene, ever the supportive partner, encouraged me to go. I packed a small bag, grabbed the few medical supplies I still had on hand, and drove down to the Astrodome, unsure of what to expect but determined to make a difference.

The scene that greeted me when I arrived was overwhelming. The Astrodome parking lot, usually empty and quiet, was now a buzzing hive of activity. Buses were arriving in droves, each one packed with evacuees from New Orleans—people who had lost everything. Volunteers, Red Cross workers, and law enforcement officers were trying to maintain some semblance of order, but the sheer number of people made it difficult. Families, clutching what few belongings they had left, stepped off the buses looking dazed and disoriented. It was as if they had escaped one nightmare only to enter another.

I made my way through the crowd and found the volunteer check-in station. After a brief introduction and a quick explanation of my medical background, I was ushered inside the Astrodome.

Inside the Astrodome: A Sea of Despair

The first thing that hit me as I walked through the doors of the Astrodome was the noise—a cacophony of voices, crying babies, people calling out for loved ones, and the general hum of thousands of displaced souls. The second thing was the smell. The air inside was thick and oppressive, a mix of sweat, stale air, and the faint odor of disinfectant. People were lying on makeshift beds—cots, blankets, even cardboard mats—spread out across the entire floor of the stadium.

I was led to a section near the edge of the stadium floor, where the Red Cross had set up a small medical area. But calling it a "medical area" was generous at best. There were no proper hospital beds, no sterile equipment, and barely any supplies. A few nurses and doctors were doing their best with what little they had, but it was clear they were in desperate need of more hands. That's where I came in.

One of the Red Cross coordinators briefed me quickly.

"We're severely understaffed," she said, looking frazzled but determined. "For now, we just need you to help bind wounds, treat minor injuries, and offer any comfort you can. Supplies are scarce, so make do with what we've got."

I nodded, feeling the weight of the task ahead. I hadn't been called "Doc" since Vietnam, but as soon as I began treating the evacuees, the familiar nickname returned. It felt strange, but in a way, it also felt right. This was what I had been trained for, all those years ago.

The First Day: Making Do

As I knelt down beside the first patient, a middle-aged woman who had cut her leg while escaping her flooded home, I realized just how ill-equipped we were. The gash on her leg was deep, but all I had was a handful of Band-Aids and some Neosporin. I cleaned the wound as best I could, applied the ointment, and covered it with multiple Band-Aids, all while apologizing for the lack of proper care.

"It's all right, Doc," she said, her voice shaky but grateful. "I'm just glad someone is here to help."

I moved on to the next patient, and the next, each story more heartbreaking than the last. Some had cuts and bruises from navigating through debris-filled floodwaters. Others were suffering from dehydration, heat exhaustion, and infections. The supplies we had were laughably inadequate, but we did what we could.

That night, after hours of treating patients, I went home exhausted but unable to shake the images of the people I had met. Their stories haunted me. One woman told me about how she and her children had spent days on the roof of their house, waiting for rescue as the floodwaters rose around them. Another man described how looters had broken into his home in the midst of the chaos, stealing what little he had left.

The stories of the floodwaters were particularly harrowing. Many of the evacuees had trudged through waist-deep water, filled with debris, sewage, and God knows what else, just to reach safety. Some had encountered snakes, others claimed to have seen alligators. The fear and uncertainty they had experienced was palpable, and I felt it was my duty to do whatever I could to help.

That night, I made a decision. I couldn't stand the thought of returning the next day with nothing but Band-Aids and Neosporin again. So, I went out and bought as many medical supplies as I could afford—bandages, antiseptic wipes, gauze, anything that might help. It wasn't much, but it was better than what we had.

The Next Day: Reinforcements Arrive

When I arrived back at the Astrodome the next morning, I was relieved to see that the situation had improved slightly. More medical personnel had arrived overnight, and the Red Cross had managed to bring in more supplies. Doctors, nurses, and EMTs from all over the country had answered the call for help. It was a comforting sight, but there was still so much work to be done.

I quickly got to work, assisting the EMTs in transporting the handicapped and disabled evacuees to other facilities within the city. The Astrodome, despite its size, couldn't accommodate everyone, and those who needed specialized care were being moved to nearby hospitals and clinics. Many of the people we transported were elderly or disabled, some in wheelchairs, others on stretchers. Their gratitude was overwhelming, and I did my best to reassure them that they were in good hands.

In the midst of the chaos, I found myself slipping back into the role of "Doc" with ease. The years I had spent as a medic in Vietnam came rushing back to me. The urgency, the need to think on my feet, to adapt to whatever situation was thrown my way—it was all so familiar. But this time, the battlefield wasn't a jungle; it was a stadium filled with people who had lost everything.

Stories of Survival

As I worked, I continued to hear the incredible stories of survival from the evacuees. One man, in his sixties, told me how he had lost his home to the floodwaters. He had tried to save as many of his belongings as he could, but in the end, all he could carry was a small bag with a few family photos and his wallet.

"It's funny," he said, his voice rough with emotion. "You spend your whole life accumulating things, and then, in a matter of hours, it's all gone. What really matters is that I'm still here, and my family's safe."

A young mother, cradling her infant daughter, spoke of the terror she had felt as the floodwaters rose around her. She had been trapped in her apartment building, unable to leave because of her baby's fragile condition.

"I didn't know what to do," she said, her eyes filling with tears. "I just prayed that someone would find us in time."

Thankfully, they had been rescued by a group of volunteers who had been going door to door in the flooded neighborhoods, searching for survivors. It was stories like these that reminded me of the strength and resilience of the human spirit, even in the face of unimaginable hardship.

A Lasting Impact

My time at the Astrodome during those weeks in the aftermath of Hurricane Katrina was an experience I will never forget. The patients I treated, the stories I heard, and the devastation I witnessed left a lasting impact on me. It was a sobering reminder of how fragile life can be, how quickly everything can change, and how important it is to offer help when it's needed most.

As I look back on that time, I am grateful that I was able to play a small part in helping the people of New Orleans during one of the darkest moments in their history. It wasn't easy—there were days when the sheer scale of the disaster felt overwhelming—but in the end, I knew that what mattered was being there, offering whatever support I could.

In the years that followed, the city of New Orleans began the slow process of rebuilding. The scars left by Katrina would never fully heal, but the resilience of the people who lived through it was a testament to the strength of the human spirit.

Chapter XIV
Reflections

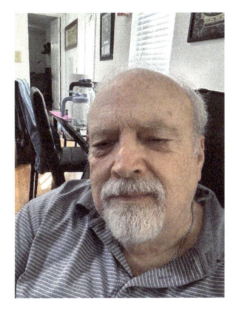

As I sit in the quiet of my home, the echoes of a life lived with purpose and pain resonate deeply within me. Looking back on my life, I find myself grappling with a complex tapestry of experiences, relationships, and emotions. I wouldn't change a thing, though. Every event, every relationship, has shaped who I am today, and I embrace it all, with both the triumphs and the trials.

The Transience of Military Life

My military experience was a crucible of transformation. When you're in the service, you form friendships and forge bonds that can be both profound and fleeting. The nature of military life is such that you move from one duty assignment to the next, leaving behind friends and allies who become like family. The relationships are intense, forged in the fires of shared experiences, but they are often strained by the very nature of the lifestyle that demands constant movement.

I learned early on to cherish the moments and to embrace the people I met, knowing full well that change was a constant companion. This ability to adapt and move on was a valuable skill, but it came with its own set of emotional costs. I would often look back on these friendships with a bittersweet sense of nostalgia, recognizing that while they enriched my life, they also left a void when they were left behind.

Childhood and Emotional Shields

Reflecting further back, I remember the deep emotional turmoil I felt as a child whenever my playmates would leave. The sense of abandonment was acute, and I would cry and feel emotionally hurt and empty. These early experiences of loss left an indelible mark on me. To cope, I built a defense mechanism, a shield around my heart. This shield, crafted in the fires of childhood pain, served me well in many respects but also prevented me from fully engaging with others later in life.

The defense mechanism I developed became a barrier, a protective wall that shielded me from emotional pain but also from the joys of deeper connections. Looking back, I see how this emotional armor, while protective, also led to isolation. Now, as I live alone, divorced and single, I can see the consequences of that shield. The walls I built to protect myself from hurt also kept me from experiencing the fullness of love and companionship.

The Strength of Service

Despite these personal challenges, I consider myself a strong individual. I answered the "call of the Trumpet," serving my country with a commitment and bravery that shaped my character. My time in the military was a formative period, one that tested my resilience and forged my sense of duty. Serving in the midst of conflict, and facing the realities of war, was a crucible that prepared me for the challenges of civilian life.

Coming home from Vietnam, I faced a new set of trials. Just two years after my return, I had to bury my parents, who perished in a fire on that fateful night in May 1977. The loss was devastating, compounded by the responsibility of helping my brother Jack care for our baby brother, who was dying of cancer during my final semester of college. The weight of these tragedies was immense, but they also served as a reminder of the strength I had developed through my military service.

Raising a Family and Facing Challenges

Raising five children and putting three of them through college, while also completing my own education, was a monumental task. The responsibilities were overwhelming, but they were also a source of immense pride. I found strength in my role as a father and provider. Each accomplishment, each milestone achieved by my children, was a testament to the love and dedication I poured into my family.

In addition to my personal responsibilities, I faced professional challenges that tested my resolve. I dared to forge ahead with innovative ideas and strategies in the retail and oil and gas industries. My career was marked by a series of bold moves and new approaches, often met with jealousy and resistance. Yet, despite the obstacles, I achieved success and found satisfaction in pushing boundaries and driving change. The rewards, particularly in the oil and gas industry, were significant enough that I chose to overlook the petty disputes and the individuals who sought to undermine my efforts.

The Struggle with Loneliness

Despite these accomplishments and the strength I drew from them, loneliness has been a persistent and challenging adversary. I tried online dating, seeking connection and companionship, but often found myself retreating before a relationship could fully develop. I would back off, squandering opportunities with many beautiful women, and at times, blocking them before they had a chance to hurt me. My old defense mechanism, the shield I had built to protect myself from emotional pain, once again reared its head.

The struggle with loneliness is a quiet and relentless battle. It creeps into the quiet moments, reminding me of the love and companionship I have pushed away. My shield, once a source of protection, has become a prison, keeping me isolated from the very connections I crave. It's a painful irony that the mechanism designed to shield me from hurt has also kept me from experiencing the joy of meaningful relationships.

Lessons from a Life Lived

Reflecting on my life, I recognize that each experience, each relationship, has been a lesson. My military service taught me discipline, resilience, and the value of camaraderie. My personal tragedies revealed the depth of human strength and the importance of perseverance. My professional experiences demonstrated the power of innovation and the ability to overcome adversity. And my struggle with loneliness has highlighted the significance of connection and vulnerability.

Life is a journey filled with highs and lows, successes and failures. Every moment, every experience, is a part of my story. A story marked by resilience, determination, and ultimately, hope. As I look ahead, I strive to live with an open heart. I seek to embrace the relationships I have and to be brave enough to form new ones. I aim to forgive myself for past mistakes and to embrace the possibilities of the future.

In the end, life is about balance. It's about finding the strength to move forward while also allowing oneself the grace to look back and reflect. It's about recognizing the lessons learned and the growth achieved. It's about living with hope and embracing the opportunities that lie ahead.

As I continue this journey, I am reminded of the strength and resilience that have carried me through. My life has been a testament to the power of perseverance and the importance of connection. I hold on to the hope that, despite the challenges, I will find the companionship and connection that have eluded me for so long. And in doing so, I will continue to write the story of my life, a story of resilience, determination, and hope.

Chapter XV
Retirement

A New Chapter Begins

After decades of dedicated service, the time had finally come for me to step away from the corporate world and begin a new chapter of my life. Apache, the company where I had spent so many years, was downsizing, and the writing was on the wall. I had seen many colleagues come and go, and now it was my turn. When the offer for a retirement package came across my desk, I knew it was the right time to accept. My official retirement date was December 31, 2019—a day that marked the end of one journey and the beginning of another.

Choosing Florida

Deciding where to spend my retirement years was not a decision I took lightly. I had always envisioned a peaceful, warm place where I could enjoy the remainder of my days. After much consideration, I chose Florida. The Sunshine State had always appealed to me with its warm climate, beautiful beaches, and relaxed lifestyle. But more than that, it was the quality of VA healthcare that ultimately swayed my decision.

As a veteran, access to quality healthcare was a top priority. The Viera VA Clinic, just 30 minutes away from my new home, was renowned for its excellent care, and the Orlando VA Hospital, only 34 minutes away, provided peace of mind that my medical needs would be well taken care of. This was crucial, given my health condition—neuropathy had left me with no feeling in my legs from my feet up to mid-thigh. While I could still drive, long distances were out of the question, so proximity to quality healthcare was essential.

But the decision to move to Florida was not just about practical considerations. My cousin Nancy, someone who had been a significant part of my life since childhood, had a condo right next to mine. The thought of living close to her again, of rekindling the close bond we had shared growing up, brought a sense of comfort and familiarity to this new phase of life.

The Journey to Florida

The move itself was no small feat. My good friend John, a steadfast companion over the years, offered to drive me from Texas to Florida. This was not just a simple favor—it was an act of deep friendship, one that I appreciated more than words can express. With neuropathy making it difficult for me to drive long distances, John's assistance was invaluable. As we drove across state lines, I couldn't help but reflect on how much my life had changed.

The journey was a mix of emotions. There was excitement about the new life awaiting me in Florida, but also a sense of melancholy as I left behind the place I had called home for so many years. Texas had been good to me, but it was time to move on. As we crossed the border into Florida, a sense of finality settled over me. This was it—my new home, my new life.

The Early Days of Retirement

Moving into my condo in Titusville was the beginning of what I hoped would be a peaceful and fulfilling retirement. The neighborhood was quiet, the weather was warm, and I had Nancy nearby for company. I spent the first few weeks settling in, getting to know the area, and making my new condo feel like home.

However, just as I was beginning to adjust to my new life, the world was hit by an unprecedented crisis—COVID-19. The pandemic swept across the globe, bringing with it fear, uncertainty, and a complete disruption of daily life. Suddenly, the retirement I had envisioned—a time of travel, socializing, and new experiences—was replaced by isolation and caution.

Life as a Hermit

COVID-19 forced many of us into a life of solitude, and for someone just beginning their retirement, the timing couldn't have been worse. The pandemic turned me into a hermit, confined to my condo, with limited interaction with the outside world. The once inviting Florida sunshine now seemed like a cruel joke, as I spent most of my days indoors, avoiding contact with others to stay safe.

The loneliness was palpable. Having moved to a new state just before the pandemic, I hadn't had the chance to build a social network or make new friends. The isolation was suffocating at times, and I found myself yearning for the company of my old friends in Houston. The retirement I had dreamed of was slipping through my fingers, replaced by a reality that I had never imagined.

A Lifeline Through Gaming

In the midst of this overwhelming loneliness, I found solace in an unexpected place—online gaming. For the past 25 years, I had been playing PC video games with my good friend Allan, and over time, our gaming group had expanded to include Marty, Bill, Bennie, Elliott, Gabe, and my son Sean. What had started as a casual hobby had become a lifeline during the pandemic.

Every evening, I would log on to my computer, connect with my friends, and lose myself in the virtual worlds of our games. It wasn't just about the games themselves—it was the camaraderie, the shared laughter, and the sense of connection that kept me going. In those moments, I wasn't just a retiree stuck in a condo in Florida—I was part of a team, engaged in adventures that took me far away from the harsh realities of the world outside.

The importance of these gaming sessions cannot be overstated. They kept me from going stir-crazy, provided a much-needed distraction from the pandemic, and helped me maintain a sense of normalcy in an otherwise abnormal time. My friendships with Allan, Marty, Bill, Bennie, Elliott, Gabe, and Sean became more vital than ever, offering a sense of community and support that I desperately needed.

Reflections on Retirement

As I reflect on my retirement journey so far, I can't help but feel a mix of emotions. There is a sense of gratitude for the life I have lived, for the opportunities I have had, and for the people who have supported me along the way. But there is also a sense of loss—loss of the retirement I had imagined, loss of the social connections I had hoped to build, and loss of the freedom to explore this new phase of life without fear.

Yet, despite these challenges, I remain hopeful. The pandemic, while difficult, has taught me valuable lessons about resilience, adaptability, and the importance of staying connected with loved ones, even if it's through a computer screen. It has reminded me that life is unpredictable, and that we must find joy and meaning wherever we can, even in the most unexpected places.

Looking Ahead

As the world slowly begins to recover from the pandemic, I am cautiously optimistic about the future. There is still much I want to do, many places I want to see, and experiences I want to have. Retirement, as I am learning, is not just about relaxation—it's about rediscovery, about finding new passions and embracing the freedom to explore them.

Florida is still new to me, and I am eager to explore all that it has to offer. I look forward to the day when I can venture out more freely, meet new people, and make the most of this new chapter in my life. The road ahead may be uncertain, but I am determined to walk it with an open heart and a spirit of adventure.

A Life Well Lived

In the end, what matters most is not where we end up, but the journey we took to get there. My journey has been filled with ups and downs, with triumphs and challenges, but through it all, I have remained true to myself. Retirement is not the end—it is simply the next step in a life well lived. And as I continue on this path, I am reminded of the words of a wise friend: "It's not about the destination, it's about the journey." And what a journey it has been.

Chapter XVI

The Weight of Legacy

As I sit down to write this final chapter, I find myself reflecting on the reasons why I started this project. It wasn't just to recount the events of my life or to document the ups and downs of my journey. It was something much deeper, something more profound. I wanted to leave behind a legacy for you, my children and grandchildren. I wanted to give you something tangible that would endure long after I'm gone—a piece of me that you can carry forward into your own lives and pass on to future generations.

This memoir is my way of sharing with you the lessons I've learned, the mistakes I've made, and the moments that have defined who I am. It's a way for me to say all the things that might have been left unsaid over the years, to express the love and pride I feel for each of you, and to acknowledge the impact you've had on my life.

Sean: The Steadfast Protector

Sean, my eldest, you have always been a rock for our family. From a young age, you demonstrated a sense of responsibility and leadership that set you apart. You were the one who stepped up when things got tough, the one who shouldered the burdens without complaint. I see so much of myself in you—my determination, my loyalty, my unwavering commitment to those I love.

I know I wasn't always the best role model, but I hope you've learned from my mistakes as well as my successes. You've grown into a strong, dependable man, and I am incredibly proud of the person you've become. Your strength, both physical and emotional, has been a source of comfort to me, and I know it will serve you well in the years to come. Keep being the protector you've always been, but don't forget to take care of yourself, too. You deserve happiness and fulfillment just as much as anyone else.

Heather: The Compassionate Healer

Heather, my dear daughter, you have a heart that is as big as the ocean. Your compassion, empathy, and kindness have always been your defining traits. From the time you were a little girl, you've had this innate ability to understand others' pain and offer comfort. It's no surprise that you chose a path in the teaching profession, dedicating your life to helping others.

You've always had a way of making people feel seen and heard, and that is a gift. I know that your journey hasn't always been easy, but you've faced every challenge with grace and resilience. I admire your strength, even when you may not see it in yourself. You've taught me so much about the power of kindness and the importance of empathy. Keep using that beautiful heart of yours to make the world a better place—you've already made mine infinitely richer.

Maria: The Fearless Explorer

Maria, my adventurous spirit, you have always been fearless in the face of the unknown. Whether it was taking on new challenges, exploring new places, or diving headfirst into new experiences, you've never been afraid to step out of your comfort zone. Your curiosity and zest for life have always inspired me.

I see in you the courage I wish I had more of when I was younger. You've taught me that life is meant to be lived fully, without fear of failure or regret. Your journey has taken you to places I could only dream of, and you've faced each new adventure with a smile on your face and a determination in your heart. I am so proud of the person you've become—strong, independent, and unafraid to chase your dreams. Keep exploring, keep pushing boundaries, and never lose that sense of wonder that makes you who you are.

Anna: The Nurturer

Anna, my sweet, gentle soul, you have always had a natural ability to care for others. Your nurturing spirit and your ability to bring people together are qualities that I have always admired. You've been the glue that holds us all together, the one who makes sure everyone is okay, even when you're struggling yourself.

Your love for your family is evident in everything you do, and it's a love that has brought us all closer together. You've shown me the importance of connection, of being there for the people you love, even when it's difficult. I know that life hasn't always been easy for you, but you've handled every obstacle with grace and strength. I am so proud of the woman you've become, and I am grateful for the love and care you've shown me and our family. Keep nurturing, keep loving, and know that you are deeply appreciated.

Marc: The Free Spirit

Marc, you have always marched to the beat of your own drum. Your creativity, your individuality, and your refusal to conform to anyone else's expectations have always set you apart. You've never been afraid to be yourself, and that is something I admire greatly.

You've taught me the value of authenticity, of being true to oneself no matter what others may think. Your journey hasn't always been easy, but you've faced every challenge with courage and a sense of humor that has kept you grounded. I am so proud of the man you've become—creative, independent, and true to yourself. Keep being the unique, wonderful person you are, and never let anyone dim your light.

To My Grandkids: Andrew and Nezelle

Andrew and Nezelle, you are the future of our family, the ones who will carry forward the legacy that your parents and I have built. You bring so much joy and light into our lives, and I am so grateful to be your grandfather.

Andrew, you have a spirit that is wise beyond your years. You're thoughtful, inquisitive, and always eager to learn. I see in you the seeds of greatness, and I know that you will achieve incredible things in your life. Keep asking questions, keep exploring, and never lose that sense of curiosity that drives you.

Nezelle, my sweet grandchild, you have a heart that is pure and full of love. You have a way of making everyone around you feel special, and that is a gift that will take you far in life. Keep spreading kindness wherever you go and know that you are loved more than words can express.

Reflections on Fatherhood

As I look back on my years as a father, I can't help but feel a mix of emotions. I know I wasn't always the perfect father—there were times when I made mistakes, times when I let you down, and times when I didn't live up to the expectations I set for myself. But through it all, my love for each of you has been unwavering. I may not have always shown it in the ways that I should have, but I hope you know how deeply I care for each of you.

Fatherhood has been one of the most challenging and rewarding experiences of my life. It has taught me patience, humility, and the importance of unconditional love. It has shown me that being a parent is not about being perfect, but about being present, about showing up even when it's hard, and about loving your children for who they are, not who you want them to be.

A Legacy of Loyalty and Fortitude

As I write this, I can see the traits that define our family—loyalty, fortitude, and a fierce determination to overcome whatever life throws our way. These are qualities that have been passed down through the generations, and I see them reflected in each of you. I am proud to be called your father, and I am even prouder of the people you have become.

You have each blazed your own paths, created your own lives, and built your own legacies. I am thankful that I have been able to witness your growth, to see you mature into the incredible adults you are today. You have taught me so much, and I am a better person because of each of you.

Lessons Learned

Writing this memoir has been a journey of self-discovery. It has forced me to confront my past, to examine my choices, and to reflect on the lessons I've learned along the way. I have come to understand that life is not about perfection—it's about progress. It's about learning from our mistakes, growing from our experiences, and always striving to be better.

I hope that this memoir will serve as a reminder to you all that it's okay to make mistakes, it's okay to stumble, and it's okay to have moments of doubt. What matters is how you respond, how you pick yourself up, and how you move forward. I hope that my story will inspire you to live your lives with courage, with integrity, and with a deep sense of purpose. Always remember the immortal words of that great sage W.C. Fields: "There comes a time in the affairs of men when one must take the bull by the tail and face the situation".

Cherishing the Memories

As I move forward into the next phase of my life, I do so with a heart full of gratitude and love for each of you. I will cherish the memories we've created together, the laughter we've shared, and the challenges we've overcome. These memories are the foundation of our family, and they will continue to be a source of strength and comfort for me in the years to come.

I want you to know that no matter where life takes you, no matter what challenges you may face, you will always have a father who loves you, who believes in you, and who is proud of you. My hope is that you will carry these memories with you, that you will draw strength from them, and that you will continue to build on the legacy that we have created together.

A Father's Love

In closing, I want to leave you with this: I love you all more than words can express. You are my greatest accomplishments, my pride, and my joy. I may not have been the perfect father, but I have always loved you with all my heart. I hope that this memoir will serve as a testament to that love and as a reminder that, no matter what, you will always have a father who loves you.

Thank you for being my children, for giving me the privilege of being your father, and for filling my life with love, laughter, and meaning. I am grateful for each of you, and I will carry that gratitude with me always.

I LOVE YOU GUYS!!

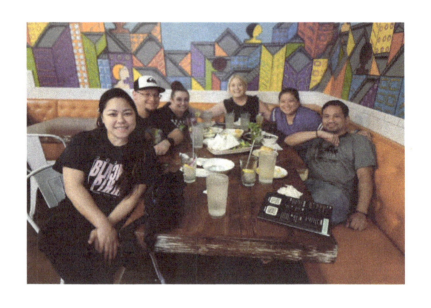